Bullous Pemphigoid Unveiled

A Comprehensive Guide

Ethan D. Anderson

Xspurts.com

A New Zealand Designed Product

Other Versions Available

Why limit yourself to just one format?

This book is now available in physical, digital, and audiobook options.

Choose the way you love to read and dive into the story today. You won't regret it!

Digital ISBN: 9781776967995
Physical ISBN: 9781776967988
Audio ISBN:

To obtain a different format of this book at a discounted price, please get in touch with us at:

http://isbn.xspurts.com/

Contents

Have Questions / Comments?

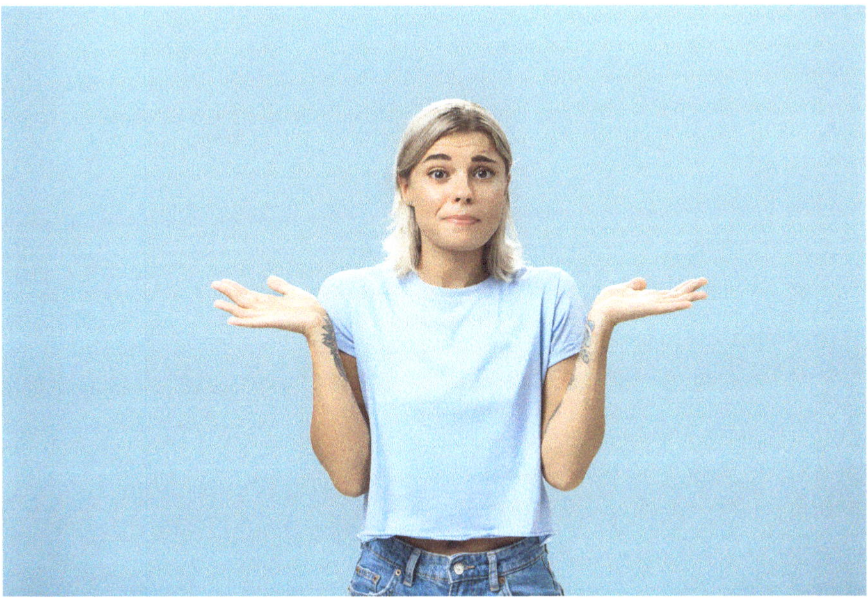

This book was designed to cover as much information as possible, but I know I have probably missed something, or some new amazing discovery has just come out.

If you notice something missing or have a question that I failed to answer, please get in touch and let me know. If I can, I will email you an answer and also update the book so others can also benefit from it.

Thanks For Being Awesome :)

Submit Your Questions / Comments At:

https://questions.xspurts.com

Get Free Stuff

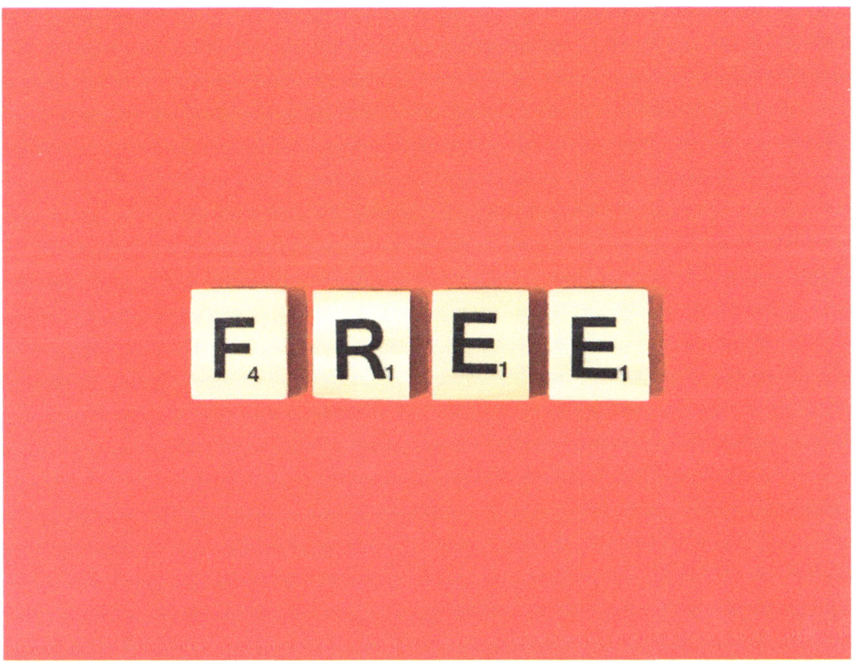

We love writing and have produced a huge number of books.

For being one of our amazing readers, we would love to offer you more books we have created, 100% free.

To claim this limited time special offer, simply go to the site below and enter your name and email address.

You will then receive loads (as we love our readers so much :) of our great books, content and audio direct to your email account, 100% free!

Get Loads of FREE Stuff at:

https://free.xspurts.com

Chapter One

Understanding Bullous Pemphigoid

Bullous pemphigoid is a rare autoimmune disorder that affects the skin and mucous membranes. It is characterized by the formation of large, fluid-filled blisters that can occur anywhere on the body. This condition is most common in older adults, and although it is not life-threatening, it can be quite uncomfortable and may require ongoing treatment.

To understand bullous pemphigoid, it's helpful to first understand the basics of the immune system. The immune system is responsible for protecting the body against foreign invaders such as viruses and bacteria. In people with bullous pemphigoid, the immune system mistakenly attacks healthy cells in the skin and mucous membranes. Specifically, it targets a protein called BP180 that is found in the skin's basement membrane.

The exact cause of bullous pemphigoid is not fully understood, but it is believed to be a combination of genetic and environmental factors. Certain medications, infections, and other autoimmune disorders may also trigger the condition.

Symptoms of bullous pemphigoid can vary from person to person, but the hallmark sign is the appearance of large, fluid-filled blisters. These blisters are often accompanied by redness, itching, and other signs of inflammation. In some cases, the blisters may break open and form open sores, which can increase the risk of infection.

Diagnosing bullous pemphigoid typically involves a combination of physical exam, biopsy, and blood tests. A skin biopsy involves removing a small sample of skin tissue for examination under a microscope. Blood tests can detect the presence of antibodies that target BP180, which can confirm the diagnosis.

Treatment for bullous pemphigoid typically involves a combination of medications and other supportive measures. The goal of treatment is to reduce inflammation and prevent further blistering. Topical and oral corticosteroids are commonly used to reduce inflammation and speed up the healing process. Other medications that may be used include immunosuppressants, antibiotics, and antihistamines.

In addition to medications, there are several other steps that people with bullous pemphigoid can take to manage their symptoms. These include keeping the skin clean and dry, avoiding irritating clothing and fabrics, and avoiding activities that can cause excessive sweating or friction on the skin. It's also important to protect the skin from sun exposure, as this can trigger flare-ups.

While bullous pemphigoid is a chronic condition that can be challenging to manage, there are several promising new treatments on the horizon. Researchers are currently exploring the use of biologic medications that target specific immune system molecules involved in the development of the condition. These medications may offer a more targeted and effective approach to treatment, with fewer side effects than traditional medications.

In addition to medical treatment, many people with bullous pemphigoid find it helpful to connect with others who have the condition. Support groups and online forums can provide a sense of community and offer practical advice for managing symptoms and coping with the emotional impact of the condition.

Definition and overview

Bullous pemphigoid is a rare autoimmune disorder that affects the skin and mucous membranes. It is characterized by the formation of large, fluid-filled blisters that can occur anywhere on the body. This condition is most common in older adults, and although it is not life-threatening, it can be quite uncomfortable and may require ongoing treatment.

To understand bullous pemphigoid, it's helpful to first understand the basics of the immune system. The immune system is responsible for protecting the body against foreign invaders such as viruses and bacteria. In people with bullous pemphigoid, the immune system mistakenly attacks healthy cells in the skin and mucous membranes. Specifically, it targets a protein called BP180 that is found in the skin's basement membrane.

The exact cause of bullous pemphigoid is not fully understood, but it is believed to be a combination of genetic and environmental factors. Certain medications, infections, and other autoimmune disorders may also trigger the condition.

Symptoms of bullous pemphigoid can vary from person to person, but the hallmark sign is the appearance of large, fluid-filled blisters. These blisters are often accompanied by redness, itching, and other signs of inflammation. In some cases, the blisters may break open and form open sores, which can increase the risk of infection.

Diagnosing bullous pemphigoid typically involves a combination of physical exam, biopsy, and blood tests. A skin biopsy involves removing a small sample of skin tissue for examination under a microscope. Blood tests can detect the presence of antibodies that target BP180, which can confirm the diagnosis.

Treatment for bullous pemphigoid typically involves a combination of medications and other supportive measures. The goal of treatment is to reduce inflammation and prevent further blistering. Topical and oral corticosteroids are commonly used to reduce inflammation and speed up the healing process. Other medications that may be used include immunosuppressants, antibiotics, and antihistamines.

In addition to medications, there are several other steps that people with bullous pemphigoid can take to manage their symptoms. These include keeping the skin clean and dry, avoiding irritating clothing and fabrics, and avoiding activities that can cause excessive sweating or friction on the skin. It's also important to protect the skin from sun exposure, as this can trigger flare-ups.

While bullous pemphigoid is a chronic condition that can be challenging to manage, there are several promising new treatments on the horizon. Researchers are currently exploring the use of biologic medications that target specific immune system molecules involved in the development of the condition. These medications may offer a more targeted and effective approach to treatment, with fewer side effects than traditional medications.

In addition to medical treatment, many people with bullous pemphigoid find it helpful to connect with others who have the condition. Support groups and online forums can provide a sense of community and offer practical advice for managing symptoms and coping with the emotional impact of the condition.

Types of pemphigoid

Pemphigoid is a group of autoimmune disorders that affect the skin and mucous membranes. These conditions are characterized by the formation of fluid-filled blisters that can occur anywhere on the body. There are several types of pemphigoid, each with its own unique set of symptoms and treatment options. In this article, we will focus on bullous pemphigoid, the most common type of pemphigoid.

Bullous pemphigoid is a chronic autoimmune disorder that primarily affects older adults. It occurs when the immune system attacks the skin's basement membrane, resulting in the formation of large, fluid-filled blisters. The blisters are typically itchy and can be quite painful, and they may be accompanied by other signs of inflammation, such as redness and swelling.

There are several subtypes of bullous pemphigoid, each with its own unique characteristics. These include:

1. Classic bullous pemphigoid: This is the most common subtype of bullous pemphigoid. It typically affects older adults and is characterized by the formation of large, tense blisters on the skin and mucous membranes.

2. Childhood bullous pemphigoid: This subtype of bullous pemphigoid primarily affects children and adolescents. It is characterized by the formation of blisters on the trunk and extremities, as well as the mucous membranes of the mouth and eyes.

3. Gestational pemphigoid: This subtype of bullous pemphigoid occurs during pregnancy and typically resolves after delivery. It is characterized by the formation of blisters on the skin and mucous membranes, as well as the development of itchy, red patches on the skin.

4. Cicatricial pemphigoid: This subtype of bullous pemphigoid primarily affects the mucous membranes of the eyes, nose, and mouth. It is charac-

terized by the formation of blisters and scarring that can lead to vision loss or other complications.

Diagnosing bullous pemphigoid typically involves a combination of physical exam, biopsy, and blood tests. A skin biopsy involves removing a small sample of skin tissue for examination under a microscope. Blood tests can detect the presence of antibodies that target the skin's basement membrane, which can confirm the diagnosis.

Treatment for bullous pemphigoid typically involves a combination of medications and other supportive measures. The goal of treatment is to reduce inflammation and prevent further blistering. Topical and oral corticosteroids are commonly used to reduce inflammation and speed up the healing process. Other medications that may be used include immunosuppressants, antibiotics, and antihistamines.

In addition to medications, there are several other steps that people with bullous pemphigoid can take to manage their symptoms. These include keeping the skin clean and dry, avoiding irritating clothing and fabrics, and avoiding activities that can cause excessive sweating or friction on the skin. It's also important to protect the skin from sun exposure, as this can trigger flare-ups.

While bullous pemphigoid is a chronic condition that can be challenging to manage, there are several promising new treatments on the horizon. Researchers are currently exploring the use of biologic medications that target specific immune system molecules involved in the development of the condition. These medications may offer a more targeted and effective approach to treatment, with fewer side effects than traditional medications.

In addition to medical treatment, many people with bullous pemphigoid find it helpful to connect with others who have the condition. Support groups and online forums can provide a sense of community and offer practical advice for managing symptoms and coping with the emotional impact of the condition.

Causes and risk factors

Bullous pemphigoid is an autoimmune disorder that causes large, fluid-filled blisters to form on the skin and mucous membranes. While the exact cause of bullous pemphigoid is not fully understood, there are several risk factors and potential triggers that may contribute to the development of the condition.

One of the primary risk factors for bullous pemphigoid is age. This condition is most common in older adults, with the average age of onset being around 70 years old. This may be due in part to changes in the immune system that occur as we age, which can make us more susceptible to autoimmune disorders like bullous pemphigoid.

In addition to age, there are several other risk factors that may increase the likelihood of developing bullous pemphigoid. These include:

1. Genetics: Like many autoimmune disorders, bullous pemphigoid appears to have a genetic component. Certain genetic variations may increase the risk of developing the condition, although more research is needed to fully understand the relationship between genetics and bullous pemphigoid.

2. Medications: Some medications may trigger an autoimmune response that leads to the development of bullous pemphigoid. These medications include antibiotics, diuretics, and certain anti-inflammatory drugs.

3. Infections: Infections can also trigger an autoimmune response that leads to the development of bullous pemphigoid. This may be because the

immune system becomes overactive in response to the infection, causing it to attack healthy cells in the skin and mucous membranes.

4. Other autoimmune disorders: People with other autoimmune disorders, such as rheumatoid arthritis or lupus, may be more likely to develop bullous pemphigoid.

5. Exposure to ultraviolet (UV) radiation: Exposure to UV radiation from the sun or tanning beds may trigger or worsen bullous pemphigoid symptoms in some people.

While these risk factors may increase the likelihood of developing bullous pemphigoid, it's important to note that many people with the condition have no known risk factors or triggers. This highlights the complex nature of autoimmune disorders and the need for further research to better understand the underlying causes and risk factors.

If you are concerned about your risk of developing bullous pemphigoid, it's important to talk to your healthcare provider. They can help you understand your individual risk factors and provide guidance on how to minimize your risk or manage the condition if you are already affected.

In addition to medical treatment, there are several lifestyle factors that may help reduce the risk of developing bullous pemphigoid or manage symptoms if you have the condition. These include:

6. Protecting your skin from UV radiation: This can be done by wearing protective clothing, using sunscreen, and avoiding direct sunlight during peak hours.

7. Eating a healthy, balanced diet: A diet rich in fruits, vegetables, whole grains, and lean protein sources may help support overall immune system health.

8. Managing stress: Stress can exacerbate autoimmune disorders like bullous pemphigoid, so finding ways to manage stress, such as through meditation or yoga, may be helpful.

9. Avoiding known triggers: If you have identified specific triggers that exacerbate your symptoms, such as certain medications or fabrics, it's important to avoid them as much as possible.

Chapter Two

Symptoms and Diagnosis

Bullous pemphigoid is an autoimmune disorder that causes large, fluid-filled blisters to form on the skin and mucous membranes. These blisters can be quite uncomfortable and may be accompanied by other signs of inflammation, such as redness, itching, and swelling. In this article, we will explore the symptoms of bullous pemphigoid and the diagnostic process used to identify the condition.

Symptoms of Bullous Pemphigoid

The symptoms of bullous pemphigoid can vary from person to person, but the hallmark sign is the appearance of large, fluid-filled blisters. These blisters can occur anywhere on the body but are most commonly found on the arms, legs, and trunk. In some cases, the blisters may be accompanied by other signs of inflammation, such as redness, itching, and swelling.

As the blisters begin to heal, they may break open and form open sores, which can increase the risk of infection. Some people with bullous pemphigoid may also develop small, raised red or pink patches on the skin, known as urticarial lesions.

In addition to skin symptoms, bullous pemphigoid can also affect the mucous membranes, such as those in the mouth, nose, and eyes. This can cause a range of symptoms, including:

Painful sores or blisters in the mouth or throat

Difficulty swallowing or eating

Redness and inflammation in the eyes

Blurred vision or vision loss

It's important to note that the symptoms of bullous pemphigoid can be similar to other skin conditions, such as herpes or dermatitis, so it's important to see a healthcare provider for a proper diagnosis.

Diagnosing Bullous Pemphigoid

Diagnosing bullous pemphigoid typically involves a combination of physical exam, biopsy, and blood tests. During the physical exam, a healthcare provider will examine the skin and mucous membranes for signs of blisters, inflammation, and other symptoms.

A skin biopsy involves removing a small sample of skin tissue for examination under a microscope. This can help confirm the presence of bullous pemphigoid and rule out other skin conditions.

Blood tests can also be used to diagnose bullous pemphigoid. Specifically, these tests can detect the presence of antibodies that target the skin's basement membrane, which is a hallmark of the condition. However, it's important to note that some people with bullous pemphigoid may have negative blood test results, so a skin biopsy is often necessary for a definitive diagnosis.

In addition to these tests, a healthcare provider may also order other diagnostic tests to rule out other conditions that can cause similar symptoms, such as herpes or dermatitis.

If you have been diagnosed with bullous pemphigoid, it's important to work closely with a healthcare provider to develop a comprehensive treatment plan. Treatment typically involves a combination of medications and other supportive measures, such as keeping the skin clean and dry and avoiding triggers that can exacerbate symptoms.

Life expectancy

Bullous pemphigoid is a chronic autoimmune disorder that causes large, fluid-filled blisters to form on the skin and mucous membranes. While bullous pemphigoid can be uncomfortable and require ongoing treatment, it typically does not significantly impact life expectancy.

That being said, there are several factors that can influence life expectancy in people with bullous pemphigoid. These include:

1. Age: As with many health conditions, age can be a significant factor in life expectancy for people with bullous pemphigoid. Older adults may be more likely to experience complications from the condition, such as infections or complications related to treatment.

2. Disease severity: The severity of bullous pemphigoid can vary from person to person, with some people experiencing milder symptoms and others experiencing more severe blistering and inflammation. In general, people with more severe cases of bullous pemphigoid may be more likely to experience complications and may have a slightly shorter life expectancy than those with milder cases.

3. Treatment: The medications used to treat bullous pemphigoid can have side effects and may increase the risk of certain complications, such as infections. In rare cases, severe complications from treatment can occur, which may impact life expectancy.

4. Co-existing health conditions: People with bullous pemphigoid may also have other health conditions that can impact life expectancy. For example, people with bullous pemphigoid may be more likely to have other

autoimmune disorders or to develop complications related to age, such as cardiovascular disease or cancer.

It's important to note that bullous pemphigoid is a chronic condition that requires ongoing management, and people with the condition should work closely with their healthcare provider to develop a comprehensive treatment plan. This may include medications to manage symptoms, such as corticosteroids or immunosuppressants, as well as lifestyle changes to minimize triggers and manage symptoms, such as avoiding sun exposure and practicing good skin hygiene.

In addition to medical treatment, many people with bullous pemphigoid find it helpful to connect with others who have the condition. Support groups and online forums can provide a sense of community and offer practical advice for managing symptoms and coping with the emotional impact of the condition.

Recognizing bullous pemphigoid symptoms

Bullous pemphigoid is an autoimmune disorder that causes large, fluid-filled blisters to form on the skin and mucous membranes. While the condition can be uncomfortable and require ongoing management, early detection and treatment can help prevent complications and improve outcomes. In this article, we will explore how to recognize the symptoms of bullous pemphigoid.

Skin Symptoms of Bullous Pemphigoid

The most common symptom of bullous pemphigoid is the appearance of large, fluid-filled blisters on the skin. These blisters can occur anywhere on the body but are most commonly found on the arms, legs, and trunk. In some cases, the blisters may be accompanied by other signs of inflammation, such as redness, itching, and swelling.

As the blisters begin to heal, they may break open and form open sores, which can increase the risk of infection. In addition to blisters, some people with bullous pemphigoid may develop small, raised red or pink patches on the skin, known as urticarial lesions.

Mucous Membrane Symptoms of Bullous Pemphigoid

In addition to skin symptoms, bullous pemphigoid can also affect the mucous membranes, such as those in the mouth, nose, and eyes. This can cause a range of symptoms, including:

Painful sores or blisters in the mouth or throat

Difficulty swallowing or eating

Redness and inflammation in the eyes

Blurred vision or vision loss

These symptoms can be particularly concerning, as they can impact daily activities such as eating and vision. If you are experiencing any of these symptoms, it's important to see a healthcare provider for an evaluation.

Diagnosis and Treatment of Bullous Pemphigoid

Diagnosing bullous pemphigoid typically involves a combination of physical exam, biopsy, and blood tests. During the physical exam, a healthcare provider will examine the skin and mucous membranes for signs of blisters, inflammation, and other symptoms.

A skin biopsy involves removing a small sample of skin tissue for examination under a microscope. This can help confirm the presence of bullous pemphigoid and rule out other skin conditions.

Blood tests can also be used to diagnose bullous pemphigoid. Specifically, these tests can detect the presence of antibodies that target the skin's basement membrane, which is a hallmark of the condition.

Once diagnosed, treatment for bullous pemphigoid typically involves a combination of medications and other supportive measures. Medications used to treat bullous pemphigoid may include corticosteroids, immunosuppressants, and other medications that help manage symptoms and reduce inflammation. In addition to medical treatment, it's important to practice good skin hygiene, avoid triggers that can exacerbate symptoms, and seek regular follow-up care with a healthcare provider.

Diagnostic tests and procedures

Bullous pemphigoid is an autoimmune disorder that causes large, fluid-filled blisters to form on the skin and mucous membranes. While the symptoms of bullous pemphigoid can be similar to other skin conditions, several diagnostic tests and procedures can help identify the condition and rule out other potential causes. In this article, we will explore the diagnostic tests and procedures used to diagnose bullous pemphigoid.

Physical Exam

A physical exam is often the first step in diagnosing bullous pemphigoid. During the exam, a healthcare provider will examine the skin and mucous membranes for signs of blisters, inflammation, and other symptoms. They may also ask about medical history, including any medications or supplements that the person is taking.

Skin Biopsy

A skin biopsy involves removing a small sample of skin tissue for examination under a microscope. This can help confirm the presence of bullous pemphigoid and rule out other skin conditions that may have similar symptoms. During the procedure, a healthcare provider will use a local anesthetic to numb the skin, then use a small, circular blade or a punch tool to remove a small piece of tissue. The tissue is then sent to a laboratory for analysis.

Blood Tests

Blood tests can also be used to diagnose bullous pemphigoid. Specifically, these tests can detect the presence of antibodies that target the skin's basement membrane, which is a hallmark of the condition. However, it's important to note that some people with bullous pemphigoid may have negative blood test results, so a skin biopsy is often necessary for a definitive diagnosis.

Direct Immunofluorescence

Direct immunofluorescence is a procedure used to identify the presence of antibodies in skin tissue samples. During the procedure, a healthcare provider will apply a fluorescent dye to a small skin sample taken from a blister or other affected area. The dye will bind to any antibodies present, which can then be viewed under a microscope. This can help confirm the presence of bullous pemphigoid and rule out other skin conditions.

Indirect Immunofluorescence

Indirect immunofluorescence is a blood test that can detect the presence of antibodies that target the skin's basement membrane. During the test, a small sample of blood is drawn from the person's arm and sent to a laboratory for analysis. If antibodies are present, the test can help confirm the presence of bullous pemphigoid.

Treatment and Management

Once diagnosed with bullous pemphigoid, treatment typically involves a combination of medications and other supportive measures. Medications used to treat bullous pemphigoid may include corticosteroids, immunosuppressants, and other medications that help manage symptoms and reduce inflammation. In addition to medical treatment, it's important to practice good skin hygiene, avoid triggers that can exacerbate symptoms, and seek regular follow-up care with a healthcare provider.

Differential diagnosis

Bullous pemphigoid is an autoimmune disorder that causes large, fluid-filled blisters to form on the skin and mucous membranes. While the symptoms of bullous pemphigoid can be similar to other skin conditions, several differential diagnoses should be considered when evaluating a person with suspected bullous pemphigoid. In this article, we will explore the differential diagnosis of bullous pemphigoid.

Pemphigus Vulgaris

Pemphigus vulgaris is another autoimmune disorder that causes blistering of the skin and mucous membranes. However, pemphigus vulgaris typically causes smaller, more fragile blisters that are more likely to break open and form painful sores. Additionally, pemphigus vulgaris tends to affect the mucous membranes more severely than the skin, while bullous pemphigoid affects both equally.

Dermatitis Herpetiformis

Dermatitis herpetiformis is a chronic skin condition that causes small, itchy blisters to form on the skin. While the blisters in dermatitis herpetiformis are smaller than those in bullous pemphigoid, they can be just as uncomfortable and may leave scars when they heal. Dermatitis herpetiformis is also associated with gluten intolerance and is often seen in people with celiac disease.

Epidermolysis Bullosa Acquisita

Epidermolysis bullosa acquisita is a rare autoimmune disorder that causes blistering of the skin and mucous membranes. However, epidermolysis bullosa acquisita tends to affect the skin more severely than the mucous membranes, and the blisters are often triggered by trauma or friction to the skin. Additionally, epidermolysis bullosa acquisita is often associated with scarring and deformities of the skin and nails.

Pemphigoid Gestationis

Pemphigoid gestationis is a rare autoimmune disorder that occurs during pregnancy and causes blistering of the skin and mucous membranes. While the symptoms of pemphigoid gestationis are similar to those of bullous pemphigoid, pemphigoid gestationis tends to be more severe and is often accompanied by intense itching. Pemphigoid gestationis typically resolves after delivery but may recur in subsequent pregnancies.

Infectious Diseases

Several infectious diseases can cause blistering of the skin and mucous membranes, including herpes simplex virus, herpes zoster virus, and varicella-zoster virus. While the blisters caused by these viruses may be similar in appearance to those seen in bullous pemphigoid, they are typically smaller and more widespread. Additionally, these viruses are often accompanied by other symptoms, such as fever and malaise.

Drug Reactions

Certain medications can cause blistering of the skin and mucous membranes as a side effect, including antibiotics, nonsteroidal anti-inflammatory drugs (NSAIDs), and anticonvulsants. While the blisters caused by drug reactions may be similar in appearance to those seen in bullous pemphigoid, they typically occur more suddenly and are more widespread. Additionally, drug reactions are often accompanied by other symptoms, such as fever, headache, and joint pain.

Chapter Three

The Immune System and Bullous Pemphigoid

Bullous pemphigoid is an autoimmune disorder that occurs when the body's immune system attacks the skin's basement membrane, which is the structure that attaches the skin to the underlying tissue. This leads to the formation of large, fluid-filled blisters on the skin and mucous membranes. In this article, we will explore the role of the immune system in the development of bullous pemphigoid.

Overview of the Immune System

1. The immune system is a complex network of cells, tissues, and organs that work together to protect the body against infections and other threats. The immune system is divided into two main categories: the innate immune system and the adaptive immune system.

The innate immune system provides the body with immediate, non-specific protection against a wide range of threats, such as bacteria and viruses. This system includes physical barriers, such as the skin and mucous membranes, as well as various immune cells that can identify and eliminate pathogens.

The adaptive immune system, on the other hand, is more specific and targeted. This system involves the production of antibodies and other immune cells that can recognize and target specific pathogens. The adaptive immune system also has a memory component, which allows it to recognize and respond more quickly to previously encountered pathogens.

Autoimmune Disorders and the Immune System

In autoimmune disorders like bullous pemphigoid, the immune system mistakenly identifies the body's own tissues as foreign and attacks them. In the case of bullous pemphigoid, the immune system targets the skin's basement membrane, leading to the formation of blisters.

The exact cause of autoimmune disorders is not fully understood, but it is thought to involve a combination of genetic and environmental factors. Certain genes may make a person more susceptible to autoimmune disorders, while environmental triggers such as infections, medications, and stress may trigger the onset of the disorder.

Immune Cells Involved in Bullous Pemphigoid

Several types of immune cells have been implicated in the development of bullous pemphigoid. These include:

2. B cells: B cells are a type of immune cell that produces antibodies, which can identify and target specific pathogens. In bullous pemphigoid, B cells produce antibodies that target the skin's basement membrane, leading to inflammation and blister formation.

3. T cells: T cells are another type of immune cell that play a role in the development of bullous pemphigoid. Specifically, T cells help activate B cells, which in turn produce the antibodies that target the skin's basement membrane.

4. Mast cells: Mast cells are immune cells that play a role in inflammation and allergic reactions. In bullous pemphigoid, mast cells are thought to release substances that cause inflammation and blister formation.

Treatment of Bullous Pemphigoid

Treatment of bullous pemphigoid typically involves medications that suppress the immune system, such as corticosteroids and immunosuppressants. These medications help reduce inflammation and prevent the immune system from attacking the skin's basement membrane. In addition to medication, other supportive measures may be recommended, such as wound care and pain management.

Autoimmune response

Bullous pemphigoid is an autoimmune disorder that occurs when the immune system mistakenly attacks the skin's basement membrane, which is the structure that attaches the skin to the underlying tissue. This leads to the formation of large, fluid-filled blisters on the skin and mucous membranes. In this article, we will explore the autoimmune response involved in the development of bullous pemphigoid.

Overview of Autoimmune Responses

Autoimmune responses occur when the immune system mistakenly attacks the body's own tissues as foreign. Normally, the immune system is able to distinguish between self and non-self and only attacks foreign invaders, such as bacteria and viruses. However, in autoimmune disorders, the immune system fails to recognize self and attacks the body's own tissues.

The exact cause of autoimmune disorders is not fully understood, but it is thought to involve a combination of genetic and environmental factors. Certain genes may make a person more susceptible to autoimmune disorders, while environmental triggers such as infections, medications, and stress may trigger the onset of the disorder.

Autoimmune Response in Bullous Pemphigoid

In bullous pemphigoid, the immune system mistakenly identifies the skin's basement membrane as foreign and attacks it. This leads to the formation of blisters on the skin and mucous membranes.

The immune cells involved in the autoimmune response in bullous pemphigoid include B cells, T cells, and mast cells. B cells are a type of immune cell that produces antibodies, which can identify and target specific pathogens. In bullous pemphigoid, B cells produce antibodies that target a protein called BP180, which is located in the skin's basement membrane. These antibodies cause inflammation and blister formation.

T cells are another type of immune cell that play a role in the development of bullous pemphigoid. Specifically, T cells help activate B cells, which in turn produce the antibodies that target BP180.

Mast cells are immune cells that play a role in inflammation and allergic reactions. In bullous pemphigoid, mast cells are thought to release substances that cause inflammation and blister formation.

Diagnosis and Treatment of Bullous Pemphigoid

Diagnosis of bullous pemphigoid typically involves a physical exam, skin biopsy, and blood tests to detect the presence of antibodies that target BP180. Treatment of bullous pemphigoid typically involves medications that suppress the immune system, such as corticosteroids and immunosuppressants. These medications help reduce inflammation and prevent the immune system from attacking the skin's basement membrane. In addition to medication, other supportive measures may be recommended, such as wound care and pain management.

Prevention and Management of Autoimmune Disorders

While the exact cause of autoimmune disorders is not fully understood, there are steps that can be taken to prevent and manage these conditions. These include:

1. Maintaining a healthy lifestyle: A healthy lifestyle, including a balanced diet, regular exercise, and stress management, can help support overall immune system health.

2. Avoiding triggers: Certain triggers, such as infections, medications, and stress, can trigger autoimmune responses in susceptible individuals. Avoiding or minimizing exposure to these triggers can help reduce the risk of developing an autoimmune disorder.

3. Seeking medical care: If symptoms of an autoimmune disorder are present, seeking medical care as soon as possible can help prevent complications and improve outcomes.

Role of antibodies

Bullous pemphigoid is an autoimmune disorder that occurs when the immune system mistakenly attacks the skin's basement membrane, which is the structure that attaches the skin to the underlying tissue. This leads to the formation of large, fluid-filled blisters on the skin and mucous membranes. In this article, we will explore the role of antibodies in the development of bullous pemphigoid.

Antibodies and the Immune System

Antibodies, also known as immunoglobulins, are proteins produced by the immune system that can identify and neutralize specific pathogens, such as bacteria and viruses. Antibodies are produced by B cells, which are a type of immune cell.

When the body encounters a foreign pathogen, B cells are activated and produce antibodies that are specific to that pathogen. These antibodies bind to the pathogen and mark it for destruction by other immune cells.

Role of Antibodies in Bullous Pemphigoid

In bullous pemphigoid, the immune system mistakenly identifies the skin's basement membrane as foreign and produces antibodies that target a protein called BP180, which is located in the basement membrane. These antibodies cause inflammation and blister formation.

Specifically, in bullous pemphigoid, B cells produce IgG antibodies that target BP180. These antibodies bind to BP180 and trigger an immune response that causes inflammation and blister formation.

In addition to IgG antibodies, IgE antibodies may also play a role in the development of bullous pemphigoid. IgE antibodies are typically associated with allergic reactions and are produced by mast cells, which are immune cells that play a role in inflammation and allergic reactions. In bullous pemphigoid, mast cells are thought to release IgE antibodies that target BP180 and contribute to inflammation and blister formation.

Diagnosis and Treatment of Bullous Pemphigoid

Diagnosis of bullous pemphigoid typically involves a physical exam, skin biopsy, and blood tests to detect the presence of antibodies that target BP180. Treatment of bullous pemphigoid typically involves medications that suppress the immune system, such as corticosteroids and immunosuppressants. These medications help reduce inflammation and prevent the immune system from attacking the skin's basement membrane. In addition to medication, other supportive measures may be recommended, such as wound care and pain management.

Prevention and Management of Autoimmune Disorders

While the exact cause of autoimmune disorders like bullous pemphigoid is not fully understood, there are steps that can be taken to prevent and manage these conditions. These include:

1. Maintaining a healthy lifestyle: A healthy lifestyle, including a balanced diet, regular exercise, and stress management, can help support overall immune system health.

2. Avoiding triggers: Certain triggers, such as infections, medications, and stress, can trigger autoimmune responses in susceptible individuals. Avoiding or minimizing exposure to these triggers can help reduce the risk of developing an autoimmune disorder.

3. Seeking medical care: If symptoms of an autoimmune disorder are present, seeking medical care as soon as possible can help prevent complications and improve outcomes.

Inflammation and skin damage

Bullous pemphigoid is an autoimmune disorder that occurs when the immune system mistakenly attacks the skin's basement membrane, which is the structure that attaches the skin to the underlying tissue. This leads to the formation of large, fluid-filled blisters on the skin and mucous membranes. In this article, we will explore the role of inflammation and skin damage in the development of bullous pemphigoid.

Inflammation and Autoimmune Disorders

Inflammation is a natural response of the immune system to injury or infection. When the body encounters a foreign pathogen or tissue damage, immune cells are activated and release substances that cause inflammation. Inflammation is characterized by redness, swelling, warmth, and pain.

In autoimmune disorders like bullous pemphigoid, the immune system mistakenly identifies the body's own tissues as foreign and attacks them. This leads to chronic inflammation and tissue damage. In bullous pemphigoid, the immune system attacks the skin's basement membrane, which leads to inflammation and blister formation.

Inflammation and Skin Damage in Bullous Pemphigoid

In bullous pemphigoid, the immune system produces antibodies that target a protein called BP180, which is located in the skin's basement membrane. These antibodies cause inflammation and blister formation. Specifically, the antibodies bind to BP180 and trigger an immune response that causes inflammation and damage to the basement membrane.

The inflammation and damage caused by bullous pemphigoid can lead to a range of symptoms, including redness, itching, and blistering. In severe cases, the blisters may rupture and become infected, leading to further complications.

Diagnosis and Treatment of Bullous Pemphigoid

Diagnosis of bullous pemphigoid typically involves a physical exam, skin biopsy, and blood tests to detect the presence of antibodies that target BP180. Treatment of bullous pemphigoid typically involves medications that suppress the immune system, such as corticosteroids and immunosuppressants. These medications help reduce inflammation and prevent the immune system from attacking the skin's basement membrane. In addition to medication, other supportive measures may be recommended, such as wound care and pain management.

Prevention and Management of Autoimmune Disorders

While the exact cause of autoimmune disorders like bullous pemphigoid is not fully understood, there are steps that can be taken to prevent and manage these conditions. These include:

1. Maintaining a healthy lifestyle: A healthy lifestyle, including a balanced diet, regular exercise, and stress management, can help support overall immune system health.

2. Avoiding triggers: Certain triggers, such as infections, medications, and stress, can trigger autoimmune responses in susceptible individuals. Avoiding or minimizing exposure to these triggers can help reduce the risk of developing an autoimmune disorder.

3. Seeking medical care: If symptoms of an autoimmune disorder are present, seeking medical care as soon as possible can help prevent complications and improve outcomes.

Chapter Four

Treatment Options

Bullous pemphigoid is an autoimmune disorder that occurs when the immune system mistakenly attacks the skin's basement membrane, leading to the formation of large, fluid-filled blisters on the skin and mucous membranes. Treatment of bullous pemphigoid typically involves medications that suppress the immune system and reduce inflammation. In this article, we will explore the various treatment options available for bullous pemphigoid.

Corticosteroids

Corticosteroids are a type of medication that reduce inflammation and suppress the immune system. In the treatment of bullous pemphigoid, corticosteroids are often used as the first line of treatment. These medications can be taken orally or applied topically to the affected areas of the skin. Oral corticosteroids, such as prednisone, are typically used in more severe cases of bullous pemphigoid.

While corticosteroids can be effective in reducing inflammation and blister formation, they can also have side effects, including weight gain, high blood pressure, and increased risk of infection. Long-term use of corticosteroids can also lead to osteoporosis and other health problems.

Immunosuppressants

In addition to corticosteroids, immunosuppressants may also be used to treat bullous pemphigoid. Immunosuppressants work by suppressing the immune system, which can help reduce inflammation and prevent further damage to the skin's basement membrane.

Azathioprine is an immunosuppressant that is commonly used in the treatment of bullous pemphigoid. Other immunosuppressants that may be used include mycophenolate mofetil and methotrexate. These medications can be taken orally or administered through injection.

Immunoglobulin Therapy

Immunoglobulin therapy involves the infusion of immunoglobulin, which are proteins that can neutralize specific pathogens and regulate the immune system. In the treatment of bullous pemphigoid, immunoglobulin therapy may be used in more severe cases when other treatments have been ineffective or have led to significant side effects.

Immunoglobulin therapy can be administered through intravenous infusion or subcutaneous injection. While this treatment option can be effective in reducing inflammation and blister formation, it can also be costly and may have side effects, including headache and nausea.

Wound Care and Pain Management

In addition to medication, other supportive measures may be recommended for the management of bullous pemphigoid. Wound care is important for preventing infection and promoting healing of the blisters. This may involve cleaning the affected areas of the skin, applying topical ointments, and using dressings to protect the blisters from further damage.

Pain management is also important in the treatment of bullous pemphigoid. Pain and discomfort associated with the blisters can be managed with over-the-counter pain medications or prescription pain relievers.

Corticosteroids

Corticosteroids are a class of medication that are widely used in the treatment of a variety of medical conditions. In the context of bullous pemphigoid, corticosteroids are often the first line of treatment and can be very effective in reducing inflammation and blisters. In this article, we will explore the use of corticosteroids in the treatment of bullous pemphigoid.

What are Corticosteroids?

Corticosteroids are a class of medication that mimic the effects of hormones produced by the adrenal gland. These hormones are involved in regulating many processes in the body, including inflammation, immune function, and metabolism. Corticosteroids can be naturally occurring or synthetic and are available in a variety of forms, including oral, injectable, and topical.

Corticosteroids and Inflammation

Corticosteroids are powerful anti-inflammatory medications and work by suppressing the immune system and reducing inflammation. Inflammation is a natural response of the immune system to injury or infection, but in autoimmune disorders like bullous pemphigoid, the immune system mistakenly attacks the body's own tissues, leading to chronic inflammation and tissue damage.

Corticosteroids can reduce inflammation by inhibiting the production of inflammatory cytokines and decreasing the activity of immune cells involved in inflammation. This can help reduce the symptoms of bullous pemphigoid, such as redness, swelling, and blistering.

Corticosteroids and Bullous Pemphigoid

In the treatment of bullous pemphigoid, corticosteroids are often the first line of treatment. Oral corticosteroids, such as prednisone, are commonly used in the treatment of bullous pemphigoid. These medications can be effective in reducing inflammation and blister formation, leading to improved symptoms and quality of life.

Topical corticosteroids may also be used to treat bullous pemphigoid. These medications are applied directly to the affected areas of the skin and can help reduce inflammation and itching. However, topical corticosteroids may not be effective in more severe cases of bullous pemphigoid.

Side Effects of Corticosteroids

While corticosteroids can be effective in the treatment of bullous pemphigoid, they can also have side effects, especially with long-term use. Common side effects of corticosteroids include weight gain, increased appetite, mood changes, high blood pressure, and increased risk of infection. Long-term use of corticosteroids can also lead to osteoporosis and other health problems.

To minimize the risk of side effects, corticosteroids are typically prescribed at the lowest effective dose for the shortest amount of time possible. Patients taking corticosteroids should also be closely monitored for any side effects and have regular check-ups with their healthcare provider.

Immunosuppressive medications

Immunosuppressive medications are a class of drugs that suppress the immune system and can be used in the treatment of a variety of medical conditions, including autoimmune disorders like bullous pemphigoid. In this article, we will explore the use of immunosuppressive medications in the treatment of bullous pemphigoid.

What are Immunosuppressive Medications?

Immunosuppressive medications work by suppressing the immune system and reducing inflammation. The immune system is responsible for protecting the body from foreign pathogens, but in autoimmune disorders like bullous pemphigoid, the immune system mistakenly attacks the body's own tissues, leading to chronic inflammation and tissue damage.

Immunosuppressive medications can be used to treat autoimmune disorders by suppressing the immune system and reducing inflammation. These medications can be taken orally or administered through injection and are typically prescribed by a healthcare provider.

Immunosuppressive Medications and Bullous Pemphigoid

In the treatment of bullous pemphigoid, immunosuppressive medications are often used in conjunction with corticosteroids or as an alternative treatment option. Immunosuppressive medications can help reduce inflammation and prevent further damage to the skin's basement membrane.

Azathioprine is an immunosuppressive medication that is commonly used in the treatment of bullous pemphigoid. This medication works by suppressing the activity of immune cells involved in inflammation and reducing the production of antibodies that target the skin's basement membrane.

Mycophenolate mofetil is another immunosuppressive medication that may be used in the treatment of bullous pemphigoid. This medication works by inhibiting the activity of immune cells involved in inflammation and reducing the production of antibodies that target the skin's basement membrane.

Other immunosuppressive medications that may be used in the treatment of bullous pemphigoid include methotrexate and cyclophosphamide.

These medications work by suppressing the immune system and reducing inflammation, which can help improve symptoms and quality of life.

Side Effects of Immunosuppressive Medications

While immunosuppressive medications can be effective in the treatment of bullous pemphigoid, they can also have side effects. Common side effects of immunosuppressive medications include nausea, vomiting, diarrhea, and increased risk of infection. Long-term use of these medications can also lead to an increased risk of cancer and other health problems.

To minimize the risk of side effects, immunosuppressive medications are typically prescribed at the lowest effective dose for the shortest amount of time possible. Patients taking immunosuppressive medications should also be closely monitored for any side effects and have regular check-ups with their healthcare provider.

Topical treatments

Topical treatments are medications that are applied directly to the skin and can be used in the treatment of a variety of skin conditions, including bullous pemphigoid. In this article, we will explore the use of topical treatments in the treatment of bullous pemphigoid.

What are Topical Treatments?

Topical treatments are medications that are applied directly to the skin and can be used to treat a variety of skin conditions. Topical treatments can be used in the treatment of bullous pemphigoid to help reduce inflammation and blister formation.

Topical Treatments and Bullous Pemphigoid

In the treatment of bullous pemphigoid, topical treatments can be used in conjunction with other medications, such as corticosteroids or immunosuppressive medications, or as a standalone treatment option. Topical treatments can help reduce inflammation and itching, and can be particularly useful in milder cases of bullous pemphigoid.

Topical corticosteroids are a commonly used topical treatment for bullous pemphigoid. These medications work by reducing inflammation and can help reduce blister formation and itching. Topical corticosteroids can be applied directly to the affected areas of skin and are available in a variety of strengths.

Calcineurin inhibitors are another class of topical medications that may be used in the treatment of bullous pemphigoid. These medications work by inhibiting the activity of immune cells involved in inflammation and can be effective in reducing inflammation and blister formation.

Other topical treatments that may be used in the treatment of bullous pemphigoid include topical antibiotics, which can help prevent infections in areas of broken skin, and emollients, which can help moisturize and protect the skin.

Side Effects of Topical Treatments

While topical treatments can be effective in the treatment of bullous pemphigoid, they can also have side effects. Common side effects of topical corticosteroids include thinning of the skin, discoloration, and increased risk of infection. Long-term use of these medications can also lead to systemic side effects, such as weight gain and high blood pressure.

Calcineurin inhibitors can also have side effects, including increased risk of infection and skin irritation. Patients using topical treatments should be closely monitored for any side effects and have regular check-ups with their healthcare provider.

Intravenous immunoglobulin (IVIG)

Intravenous immunoglobulin (IVIG) is a medication that can be used in the treatment of a variety of medical conditions, including autoimmune disorders like bullous pemphigoid. In this article, we will explore the use of IVIG in the treatment of bullous pemphigoid.

What is IVIG?

IVIG is a medication that contains antibodies derived from the blood plasma of thousands of donors. These antibodies can help boost the immune system and can be used to treat a variety of medical conditions, including immune deficiencies and autoimmune disorders.

IVIG and Bullous Pemphigoid

In the treatment of bullous pemphigoid, IVIG can be used as an alternative treatment option for patients who are unable to tolerate or do not respond to other treatments, such as corticosteroids or immunosuppressive medications.

IVIG works by providing the patient with a large amount of antibodies that can help regulate the immune system and reduce inflammation. IVIG can also help reduce the production of antibodies that target the skin's basement membrane, which is a hallmark of bullous pemphigoid.

IVIG is typically administered through an intravenous infusion and can take several hours to complete. Patients may receive several doses of IVIG over the course of several weeks or months, depending on their individual case and response to treatment.

Side Effects of IVIG

While IVIG can be effective in the treatment of bullous pemphigoid, it can also have side effects. Common side effects of IVIG include headache, fever, and chills. Rarely, more serious side effects can occur, such as kidney damage and allergic reactions.

To minimize the risk of side effects, patients receiving IVIG are closely monitored by healthcare providers during and after the infusion. Patients should also report any side effects to their healthcare provider immediately.

Plasmapheresis

Plasmapheresis is a medical procedure that can be used in the treatment of a variety of medical conditions, including autoimmune disorders like bullous pemphigoid. In this article, we will explore the use of plasmapheresis in the treatment of bullous pemphigoid.

What is Plasmapheresis?

Plasmapheresis is a medical procedure that involves the removal, treatment, and return of blood plasma. During plasmapheresis, blood is removed from the patient's body and passed through a machine that separates the plasma from the other components of blood, such as red and white blood cells. The plasma is then treated to remove harmful antibodies or other substances before being returned to the patient's body.

Plasmapheresis and Bullous Pemphigoid

In the treatment of bullous pemphigoid, plasmapheresis can be used as an alternative treatment option for patients who are unable to tolerate or do not respond to other treatments, such as corticosteroids or immunosuppressive medications.

Plasmapheresis works by removing the harmful antibodies that target the skin's basement membrane, which is a hallmark of bullous pemphigoid. By removing these antibodies, plasmapheresis can help reduce inflammation and blister formation.

Plasmapheresis is typically performed in a hospital or outpatient clinic setting and can take several hours to complete. Patients may receive several plasmapheresis treatments over the course of several weeks or months, depending on their individual case and response to treatment.

Side Effects of Plasmapheresis

While plasmapheresis can be effective in the treatment of bullous pemphigoid, it can also have side effects. Common side effects of plasmapheresis include low blood pressure, nausea, and fatigue. Rarely, more serious side effects can occur, such as infection and allergic reactions.

To minimize the risk of side effects, patients undergoing plasmapheresis are closely monitored by healthcare providers during and after the procedure. Patients should also report any side effects to their healthcare provider immediately.

Chapter Five

Managing Side Effects of Treatment

Bullous pemphigoid is a chronic autoimmune disorder that can be managed with various treatment options, such as corticosteroids, immunosuppressive medications, IVIG, and plasmapheresis. However, these treatments can cause side effects that can affect a patient's quality of life. In this article, we will explore how to manage the side effects of treatment for bullous pemphigoid.

Corticosteroids

Corticosteroids are a commonly used treatment option for bullous pemphigoid. However, long-term use of corticosteroids can lead to side effects such as weight gain, high blood pressure, osteoporosis, and increased risk of infections. To manage the side effects of corticosteroids, patients should follow a healthy diet and exercise regularly to maintain a healthy weight and prevent bone loss. Patients should also monitor their blood pressure regularly and work with their healthcare provider to manage any high blood pressure.

Immunosuppressive Medications

Immunosuppressive medications are another treatment option for bullous pemphigoid. These medications work by suppressing the immune system, which can lead to an increased risk of infections. Patients should take extra precautions to prevent infections, such as washing their hands regularly, avoiding contact with sick individuals, and receiving recommended vaccines.

IVIG and Plasmapheresis

IVIG and plasmapheresis are alternative treatment options for bullous pemphigoid. These treatments can cause side effects such as headaches, fever, and chills. To manage these side effects, patients should rest and stay hydrated. Patients should also report any severe or persistent side effects to their healthcare provider immediately.

Alternative Treatments

Some patients may opt for alternative treatments, such as herbal remedies or dietary supplements, to manage their symptoms. However, these treatments can also have side effects and may interact with prescription medications. Patients should speak with their healthcare provider before starting any alternative treatments.

Psychological Support

Living with bullous pemphigoid and its associated treatments can be challenging and can lead to stress and anxiety. Patients should seek support from loved ones and consider talking to a mental health professional to manage their emotional well-being.

Reducing the risk of infection

Bullous pemphigoid is a chronic autoimmune disorder that can weaken the immune system and increase the risk of infection. Patients with bullous pemphigoid should take extra precautions to reduce the risk of infection. In this article, we will explore some ways to reduce the risk of infection for patients with bullous pemphigoid.

Wash Hands Frequently

One of the most effective ways to reduce the risk of infection is to wash hands frequently. Patients should wash their hands with soap and warm water for at least 20 seconds before eating, after using the bathroom, and after touching potentially contaminated surfaces. Patients should also carry hand sanitizer with them when they are unable to wash their hands.

Avoid Contact with Sick Individuals

Patients with bullous pemphigoid should avoid close contact with individuals who have a contagious illness, such as the flu or a cold. Patients should also avoid large crowds and public places during flu season or when there is an outbreak of a contagious illness.

Practice Good Hygiene

Patients with bullous pemphigoid should practice good hygiene to reduce the risk of infection. This includes keeping wounds and blisters clean and dry, covering wounds with a sterile dressing, and avoiding sharing personal items, such as towels or razors.

Receive Recommended Vaccines

Patients with bullous pemphigoid should receive recommended vaccines to prevent infections, such as the flu vaccine and pneumonia vaccine. Patients should also consult with their healthcare provider about other recommended vaccines, such as the shingles vaccine.

Take Antibiotics as Prescribed

If a patient with bullous pemphigoid develops an infection, antibiotics may be prescribed to treat the infection. Patients should take antibiotics as prescribed and complete the entire course of antibiotics, even if they start feeling better before the course is complete.

Nutrition and Hydration

Eating a healthy diet and staying hydrated can help support the immune system and reduce the risk of infection. Patients with bullous pemphigoid should eat a diet rich in fruits, vegetables, lean protein, and whole grains. Patients should also drink plenty of water and avoid sugary drinks and alcohol.

Coping with gastrointestinal issues

Bullous pemphigoid is a chronic autoimmune disorder that can cause gastrointestinal issues, such as nausea, vomiting, diarrhea, and abdominal pain. Coping with these issues can be challenging and can affect a patient's quality of life. In this article, we will explore some ways to cope with gastrointestinal issues in patients with bullous pemphigoid.

Dietary Changes

Making dietary changes can help manage gastrointestinal issues in patients with bullous pemphigoid. Patients should avoid foods that trigger their symptoms, such as spicy or fatty foods. Patients should also eat smaller, more frequent meals and avoid eating late at night. Patients may benefit from a low-fiber diet or a low-lactose diet, depending on their individual symptoms.

Medications

Patients with bullous pemphigoid may be prescribed medications to manage their gastrointestinal symptoms, such as anti-nausea medication, antidiarrheal medication, or proton pump inhibitors to reduce stomach acid. Patients should take these medications as prescribed and report any side effects to their healthcare provider.

Hydration

Staying hydrated is important for patients with bullous pemphigoid who are experiencing gastrointestinal issues. Patients should drink plenty of water and avoid drinks that can worsen their symptoms, such as alcohol, caffeine, and sugary drinks.

Stress Management

Stress can worsen gastrointestinal symptoms in patients with bullous pemphigoid. Patients should practice stress management techniques, such as deep breathing, meditation, yoga, or counseling. Patients may also benefit from engaging in relaxing activities, such as reading, listening to music, or taking a warm bath.

Exercise

Regular exercise can help manage gastrointestinal symptoms in patients with bullous pemphigoid. Patients should aim to engage in low-impact exercise, such as walking or yoga, for at least 30 minutes per day. Patients should consult with their healthcare provider before starting any exercise program.

Probiotics

Probiotics are beneficial bacteria that can help maintain a healthy gut microbiome. Patients with bullous pemphigoid may benefit from taking probiotic supplements or consuming probiotic-rich foods, such as yogurt or kefir. Patients should consult with their healthcare provider before starting any new supplements.

Minimizing bone loss

Bullous pemphigoid is a chronic autoimmune disorder that can increase the risk of bone loss, which can lead to osteoporosis and fractures. Bone loss can be a serious complication of bullous pemphigoid and can significantly affect a patient's quality of life. In this article, we will explore some ways to minimize bone loss in patients with bullous pemphigoid.

Dietary Changes

Making dietary changes can help minimize bone loss in patients with bullous pemphigoid. Patients should consume foods that are rich in calcium and vitamin D, which are important for bone health. Calcium-rich foods include dairy products, leafy green vegetables, and fortified foods such as orange juice and cereal. Vitamin D can be found in fatty fish, egg yolks, and fortified foods such as milk and cereal. Patients should also limit their intake of caffeine and alcohol, which can increase the risk of bone loss.

Exercise

Regular exercise can help minimize bone loss in patients with bullous pemphigoid. Weight-bearing exercises, such as walking, jogging, and weightlifting, can help stimulate bone growth and reduce the risk of bone loss. Patients should aim to engage in weight-bearing exercises for at least 30 minutes per day, five days per week. Patients should consult with their healthcare provider before starting any exercise program.

Bone Density Testing

Patients with bullous pemphigoid should undergo regular bone density testing to monitor their bone health. A bone density test measures the density of bones and can identify if a patient is at risk of developing osteoporosis. Patients should discuss the appropriate timing of bone density testing with their healthcare provider.

Medications

Patients with bullous pemphigoid may be prescribed medications to minimize bone loss. Bisphosphonates are a class of medications that can reduce the risk of fractures by slowing down bone loss. Other medications, such as hormone replacement therapy or calcitonin, may also be prescribed to minimize bone loss. Patients should take these medications as prescribed and report any side effects to their healthcare provider.

Supplements

Patients with bullous pemphigoid may benefit from taking calcium and vitamin D supplements to minimize bone loss. Patients should consult with their healthcare provider before starting any new supplements.

Addressing emotional well-being

Bullous pemphigoid is a chronic autoimmune disorder that can significantly affect a patient's emotional well-being. Living with a chronic illness can be challenging, and patients with bullous pemphigoid may experience a range of emotions, including anxiety, depression, and frustration. In this article, we will explore some ways to address emotional well-being in patients with bullous pemphigoid.

Education

Education is an important part of addressing emotional well-being in patients with bullous pemphigoid. Patients should be educated about their condition, including its causes, symptoms, and treatment options. Patients should also be informed about the potential emotional impact of their condition and provided with resources and support to help them cope.

Support Groups

Support groups can be an excellent resource for patients with bullous pemphigoid. Support groups provide patients with a safe and supportive environment to share their experiences, learn from others, and receive emotional support. Patients can find support groups in their local community or online.

Counseling

Counseling can be an effective way to address emotional well-being in patients with bullous pemphigoid. Counseling can help patients to manage their emotions, develop coping strategies, and improve their overall quality of life. Patients can speak with their healthcare provider about obtaining counseling services.

Mindfulness and Relaxation Techniques

Mindfulness and relaxation techniques can be helpful in managing the emotional impact of bullous pemphigoid. These techniques can help patients to manage stress, reduce anxiety and depression, and improve overall well-being. Techniques such as deep breathing, meditation, and yoga can be effective in promoting relaxation and reducing stress.

Exercise

Regular exercise can also be beneficial for addressing emotional well-being in patients with bullous pemphigoid. Exercise can help to reduce stress and anxiety, improve mood, and promote overall well-being. Patients should aim to engage in regular exercise, such as walking or swimming, for at least 30 minutes per day, five days per week.

Medication

In some cases, medication may be prescribed to address emotional well-being in patients with bullous pemphigoid. Antidepressants or anti-anxiety medications may be prescribed to help manage symptoms of depression or anxiety. Patients should take these medications as prescribed and report any side effects to their healthcare provider.

Chapter Six

Living with Bullous Pemphigoid

Bullous pemphigoid is a chronic autoimmune disorder that can significantly impact a patient's daily life. Living with bullous pemphigoid can be challenging, but with proper management and support, patients can lead fulfilling lives. In this article, we will explore some tips for living with bullous pemphigoid.

Follow Treatment Plan

Following a treatment plan is essential for managing bullous pemphigoid. Patients should take their medications as prescribed, attend regular appointments with their healthcare provider, and undergo any necessary testing. It is important for patients to communicate any changes in their symptoms or side effects to their healthcare provider promptly.

Skin Care

Skin care is an important aspect of managing bullous pemphigoid. Patients should keep their skin clean and dry, avoid scratching or rubbing their skin, and use gentle, fragrance-free products. Patients should also avoid exposure to extreme temperatures, such as hot showers or cold weather, which can trigger flare-ups.

Diet

Diet can play a role in managing bullous pemphigoid. Patients should aim to consume a well-balanced diet that is rich in nutrients, including fruits, vegetables, whole grains, lean protein, and healthy fats. Patients should also limit their intake of processed foods, sugar, and saturated and trans fats, which can contribute to inflammation.

Exercise

Regular exercise can be beneficial for managing bullous pemphigoid. Exercise can help to reduce stress, improve mood, and promote overall well-being. Patients should aim to engage in regular exercise, such as walking or swimming, for at least 30 minutes per day, five days per week. Patients should consult with their healthcare provider before starting any exercise program.

Manage Stress

Stress can trigger flare-ups in patients with bullous pemphigoid. Patients should practice stress management techniques, such as deep breathing, meditation, and yoga, to help manage their stress levels. Patients should also prioritize self-care activities, such as spending time with loved ones or engaging in hobbies that bring them joy.

Support

Having a support system is important for managing bullous pemphigoid. Patients should seek support from family and friends, participate in support groups, and consider counseling if needed. Support can provide patients with emotional and practical support, which can help them to better manage their condition.

Daily skincare routine

For patients with bullous pemphigoid, a daily skincare routine is an essential part of managing their condition. Bullous pemphigoid can cause painful blisters and lesions on the skin, which can become infected if not properly cared for. In this article, we will explore some tips for a daily skincare routine for patients with bullous pemphigoid.

Cleanse

Cleansing the skin is an important part of a daily skincare routine for patients with bullous pemphigoid. Patients should use a gentle, fragrance-free cleanser to avoid further irritation to the skin. It is important to avoid scrubbing or rubbing the skin, as this can cause the blisters to burst and lead to infection. Patients should rinse their skin thoroughly with lukewarm water and gently pat it dry with a clean, soft towel.

Moisturize

Moisturizing the skin is an important step in a daily skincare routine for patients with bullous pemphigoid. Moisturizers can help to soothe the skin and prevent dryness, which can exacerbate symptoms of bullous pemphigoid. Patients should choose a moisturizer that is fragrance-free and non-irritating. It is important to apply moisturizer immediately after cleansing the skin to lock in moisture.

Protect

Protecting the skin from further damage is essential for patients with bullous pemphigoid. Patients should avoid exposure to extreme temperatures, such as hot showers or cold weather, which can trigger flare-ups. It is also important to wear protective clothing, such as long-sleeved shirts and hats, to prevent sun damage to the skin.

Avoid Irritants

Patients with bullous pemphigoid should avoid using products that can irritate the skin, such as harsh soaps, fragrances, and abrasive scrubs. It is also important to avoid contact with irritants, such as chemicals or harsh detergents. Patients should opt for gentle, fragrance-free products and avoid products that contain alcohol or other irritants.

Treat Blisters

If blisters do appear, it is important to treat them promptly to prevent infection. Patients should clean the affected area with a gentle cleanser and lukewarm water, and apply a non-stick, sterile dressing to the blister. Patients should avoid puncturing or popping blisters, as this can lead to infection. If blisters become infected or show signs of spreading, patients should seek medical attention.

Diet and nutrition

Bullous pemphigoid is a chronic autoimmune disorder that can be managed with a healthy lifestyle, including a balanced diet and proper nutrition. Proper nutrition can help to support the immune system, reduce inflammation, and promote overall well-being. In this article, we will explore some tips for diet and nutrition for patients with bullous pemphigoid.

Eat a Balanced Diet

A balanced diet is essential for maintaining good health and managing bullous pemphigoid. Patients should aim to consume a diet that is rich in fruits, vegetables, whole grains, lean protein, and healthy fats. These foods provide essential nutrients, including vitamins, minerals, and antioxidants, which can help to support the immune system and reduce inflammation.

Limit Processed Foods

Processed foods can be high in sugar, sodium, and unhealthy fats, which can contribute to inflammation and exacerbate symptoms of bullous pemphigoid. Patients should aim to limit their intake of processed foods and choose whole, unprocessed foods whenever possible.

Avoid Trigger Foods

Certain foods can trigger inflammation and exacerbate symptoms of bullous pemphigoid. Patients should avoid foods that they have identified as triggers, such as spicy foods, alcohol, and caffeine. Patients should also avoid foods that they are allergic or intolerant to, as these can trigger symptoms.

Choose Anti-inflammatory Foods

Certain foods have anti-inflammatory properties, which can help to reduce inflammation in the body and manage symptoms of bullous pemphigoid. Patients should choose foods that are rich in omega-3 fatty acids, such as fatty fish, nuts, and seeds. Patients should also consume foods that are high in antioxidants, such as berries, leafy greens, and citrus fruits.

Stay Hydrated

Proper hydration is essential for maintaining good health and managing bullous pemphigoid. Patients should aim to drink at least 8-10 cups of water per day to stay hydrated. Patients can also consume hydrating foods, such as watermelon and cucumber, to increase their fluid intake.

Consider Supplements

Supplements can be beneficial for patients with bullous pemphigoid, particularly those who may have nutrient deficiencies. Patients should consult with their healthcare provider before taking any supplements to ensure that they are safe and effective. Some supplements that may be beneficial for patients with bullous pemphigoid include vitamin D, vitamin B12, and probiotics.

Exercise and physical activity

Exercise and physical activity are important components of a healthy lifestyle for individuals with bullous pemphigoid. Although physical activity may seem daunting for those with bullous pemphigoid, incorporating exercise into daily life can help to improve physical health, reduce inflammation, and promote emotional well-being. In this article, we will explore the benefits of exercise for patients with bullous pemphigoid and offer tips for incorporating physical activity into daily life.

Benefits of Exercise

Exercise has been shown to provide numerous health benefits for individuals with bullous pemphigoid. Regular exercise can help to improve cardiovascular health, strengthen muscles and bones, and reduce inflammation. Exercise can also improve emotional well-being by reducing stress and anxiety and promoting relaxation. Additionally, exercise can help to improve sleep quality and promote healthy weight management.

Types of Exercise

Patients with bullous pemphigoid should aim to incorporate a variety of exercise types into their routine, including aerobic exercise, strength training, and stretching. Aerobic exercise, such as walking, jogging, or cycling, can help to improve cardiovascular health and reduce inflammation. Strength training, such as weight lifting or resistance band exercises, can help to improve muscle strength and bone density. Stretching exercises, such as yoga or Pilates, can help to improve flexibility and promote relaxation.

Considerations for Exercise

Patients with bullous pemphigoid should consult with their healthcare provider before beginning an exercise routine to ensure that it is safe and appropriate for their specific needs. Patients should also consider their current level of fitness and any physical limitations when choosing an exercise routine. It is important to start slowly and gradually increase intensity and duration over time to avoid injury or exacerbating symptoms.

Tips for Incorporating Exercise

Incorporating physical activity into daily life can be challenging, but there are several ways to make it more manageable. Patients with bullous pemphigoid should aim to find activities that they enjoy and can realistically fit into their daily routine. For example, patients can go for a walk or swim, take a yoga class, or participate in a gentle aerobics class. It is important to set realistic goals and track progress to stay motivated and engaged in the exercise routine.

Incorporating Physical Activity into Daily Life

Patients with bullous pemphigoid can incorporate physical activity into their daily routine in various ways. Patients can take the stairs instead of the elevator, park farther away from their destination to increase walking distance, or take a quick walk during their lunch break. Patients can also consider using a pedometer or fitness tracker to monitor their activity level and set goals for increasing steps or activity.

Stress management

Stress management is an important aspect of managing bullous pemphigoid. Stress can trigger or worsen symptoms of the condition, and managing stress can help to reduce inflammation, improve emotional well-being, and promote overall health. In this article, we will explore the importance of stress management for patients with bullous pemphigoid and offer tips for reducing stress and managing symptoms.

Effects of Stress on Bullous Pemphigoid

Stress can have a negative impact on individuals with bullous pemphigoid. Stress can trigger or exacerbate symptoms, including blistering and skin inflammation. Stress can also weaken the immune system and increase inflammation throughout the body, making it more difficult to manage symptoms of the condition. Additionally, stress can have negative effects on emotional well-being, leading to feelings of anxiety, depression, or isolation.

Stress Management Techniques

There are several stress management techniques that individuals with bullous pemphigoid can incorporate into their daily routine. These techniques can help to reduce stress, manage symptoms, and improve overall well-being. Some effective stress management techniques include:

1. Mindfulness Meditation: Mindfulness meditation involves focusing on the present moment and observing thoughts and feelings without judgment. This technique has been shown to reduce stress and improve emotional well-being.

2. Deep Breathing: Deep breathing exercises can help to reduce stress and promote relaxation. These exercises involve taking slow, deep breaths and exhaling slowly.

3. Yoga: Yoga is a mind-body practice that combines physical postures, breathing techniques, and meditation. Yoga can help to reduce stress and improve physical and emotional well-being.

4. Progressive Muscle Relaxation: Progressive muscle relaxation involves tensing and relaxing muscles throughout the body to promote relaxation and reduce stress.

5. Cognitive Behavioral Therapy: Cognitive behavioral therapy is a type of psychotherapy that focuses on changing negative thought patterns and behaviors. This therapy can be effective in reducing stress and managing symptoms of bullous pemphigoid.

Incorporating Stress Management Techniques into Daily Life

Patients with bullous pemphigoid can incorporate stress management techniques into their daily routine in various ways. Patients can set aside time for mindfulness meditation or deep breathing exercises each day. Patients can also participate in a yoga class or practice progressive muscle relaxation in the evenings. Additionally, patients can consider speaking with a therapist or counselor to learn cognitive behavioral therapy techniques and strategies for managing stress and improving emotional well-being.

Additional Tips for Managing Stress

In addition to incorporating stress management techniques into daily life, there are several other strategies for managing stress and promoting well-being. Patients with bullous pemphigoid should aim to get adequate sleep each night, eat a healthy and balanced diet, and engage in regular physical activity. Patients can also consider seeking social support through family, friends, or support groups.

Chapter Seven

Emotional Support and Coping Strategies

Bullous pemphigoid is a chronic autoimmune disease that can have a significant impact on an individual's emotional well-being. Coping with the physical and emotional challenges of the condition can be difficult, and emotional support and coping strategies are essential for managing the disease. In this article, we will explore the importance of emotional support and coping strategies for individuals with bullous pemphigoid and offer tips for managing the emotional aspects of the condition.

The Emotional Impact of Bullous Pemphigoid

Bullous pemphigoid can have a significant impact on an individual's emotional well-being. The chronic nature of the condition, the physical symptoms, and the potential for scarring and disfigurement can all contribute to feelings of anxiety, depression, or isolation. Additionally, the treatment for bullous pemphigoid can have side effects, including weight gain, mood changes, and increased risk of infection, which can further exacerbate emotional distress.

Emotional Support

Emotional support is an essential component of managing bullous pemphigoid. Emotional support can come from family, friends, healthcare professionals, or support groups. Support from loved ones can help to reduce feelings of isolation and provide a sense of comfort and understanding. Healthcare professionals can offer guidance and support in managing symptoms and side effects of treatment. Support groups can offer a safe and supportive environment for individuals with bullous pemphigoid to share their experiences and learn from others who are going through similar challenges.

Coping Strategies

There are several coping strategies that individuals with bullous pemphigoid can incorporate into their daily routine to manage the emotional aspects of the condition. These strategies can help to reduce stress, promote relaxation, and improve overall emotional well-being. Some effective coping strategies include:

1. Self-care: Engaging in self-care activities, such as taking a relaxing bath, practicing mindfulness, or engaging in a favorite hobby, can help to reduce stress and promote emotional well-being.

2. Journaling: Writing down thoughts and feelings in a journal can help to process emotions and reduce feelings of stress or anxiety.

3. Talk Therapy: Speaking with a therapist or counselor can help individuals with bullous pemphigoid to process emotions and develop effective coping strategies for managing the emotional aspects of the condition.

4. Physical Activity: Regular physical activity, such as walking, swimming, or yoga, can help to reduce stress and improve overall emotional well-being.

5. Relaxation Techniques: Incorporating relaxation techniques, such as deep breathing or progressive muscle relaxation, into daily routine can help to promote relaxation and reduce stress.

6. Social Support: Connecting with others who have similar experiences or participating in support groups can offer emotional support and reduce feelings of isolation.

Incorporating Coping Strategies into Daily Life

Patients with bullous pemphigoid can incorporate coping strategies into their daily routine in various ways. Patients can set aside time for self-care activities, such as taking a bath or engaging in a favorite hobby, each day. Patients can also practice journaling in the evenings or participate in talk therapy sessions as needed. Additionally, patients can engage in regular physical activity, such as taking a walk or practicing yoga, and incorporate relaxation techniques, such as deep breathing or progressive muscle relaxation, into their daily routine.

Additional Tips for Managing Emotional Well-Being

In addition to incorporating coping strategies into daily life, there are several other strategies for managing emotional well-being. Patients with bullous pemphigoid should aim to get adequate sleep each night, eat a healthy and balanced diet, and engage in regular physical activity. Patients can also consider seeking out social support through family, friends, or support groups. Additionally, patients should communicate with their healthcare team about any emotional or psychological symptoms they may be experiencing, as these symptoms may require additional support or treatment

Dealing with the psychological impact

Bullous pemphigoid is a chronic autoimmune disease that can have a significant impact on an individual's psychological well-being. The physical symptoms of the condition, including painful blisters and lesions, can be distressing and can lead to feelings of anxiety, depression, or isolation. Additionally, the treatments for bullous pemphigoid can have side effects, such as weight gain and mood changes, which can further exacerbate psychological distress. In this article, we will explore the psychological impact of bullous pemphigoid and offer tips for managing the psychological aspects of the condition.

The Psychological Impact of Bullous Pemphigoid

Bullous pemphigoid can have a significant impact on an individual's psychological well-being. The physical symptoms of the condition, including painful blisters and lesions, can be distressing and can lead to feelings of anxiety, depression, or isolation. Additionally, the treatments for bullous pemphigoid can have side effects, such as weight gain and mood changes, which can further exacerbate psychological distress.

Managing the Psychological Impact of Bullous Pemphigoid

Managing the psychological impact of bullous pemphigoid requires a holistic approach that addresses both the physical and psychological aspects of the condition. Here are some tips for managing the psychological impact of bullous pemphigoid:

1. Seek Psychological Support: Speaking with a therapist or counselor can help individuals with bullous pemphigoid to process emotions and develop effective coping strategies for managing the psychological aspects of the condition. A therapist can also provide support in managing stress and anxiety related to the condition.

2. Connect with Others: Connecting with others who have similar experiences or participating in support groups can offer emotional support and reduce feelings of isolation. Consider joining a local support group or an online community dedicated to individuals with bullous pemphigoid.

3. Practice Mindfulness: Practicing mindfulness, such as meditation or yoga, can help individuals with bullous pemphigoid to manage stress and anxiety related to the condition. Mindfulness can also promote overall psychological well-being.

4. Engage in Self-Care: Engaging in self-care activities, such as taking a relaxing bath, practicing mindfulness, or engaging in a favorite hobby, can help to reduce stress and promote psychological well-being.

5. Practice Positive Self-Talk: Positive self-talk can help individuals with bullous pemphigoid to maintain a positive outlook and reduce feelings of anxiety or depression. Consider using positive affirmations or visualizations to help promote positive self-talk.

6. Communicate with Healthcare Team: Patients should communicate with their healthcare team about any psychological symptoms they may be experiencing, as these symptoms may require additional support or treatment.

Incorporating Psychological Support into Daily Life

Patients with bullous pemphigoid can incorporate psychological support strategies into their daily routine in various ways. Patients can set aside time for self-care activities, such as taking a bath or engaging in a favorite hobby, each day. Patients can also practice mindfulness in the mornings or participate in talk therapy sessions as needed. Additionally, patients can engage in regular physical activity, such as taking a walk or practicing yoga, and incorporate positive self-talk and affirmations into their daily routine.

Additional Tips for Managing Psychological Well-Being

In addition to incorporating psychological support into daily life, there are several other strategies for managing psychological well-being. Patients with bullous pemphigoid should aim to get adequate sleep each night, eat a healthy and balanced diet, and engage in regular physical activity. Patients can also consider seeking out social support through family, friends, or support groups. Additionally, patients should communicate with their healthcare team about any psychological symptoms they may be experiencing, as these symptoms may require additional support or treatment.

Building a support network

Building a strong support network is an essential part of managing any chronic illness, including bullous pemphigoid. A support network can provide emotional support, practical assistance, and a sense of community for individuals with bullous pemphigoid. In this article, we will discuss the importance of building a support network and offer tips for creating and maintaining a support network.

The Importance of Building a Support Network for Bullous Pemphigoid

Bullous pemphigoid can be a challenging condition to manage, both physically and emotionally. It can be helpful to have a support network in place to provide emotional support, practical assistance, and a sense of community. A support network can include family members, friends, healthcare professionals, and support groups.

Family and Friends

Family members and friends can be a crucial source of support for individuals with bullous pemphigoid. They can provide emotional support, help with daily tasks, and offer a sense of normalcy during difficult times. Family and friends can also provide a listening ear and offer practical solutions to challenges that may arise.

Healthcare Professionals

Healthcare professionals can provide medical treatment and support for individuals with bullous pemphigoid. They can also offer information about the condition, help manage symptoms, and provide guidance on lifestyle changes that may help to improve overall health. Healthcare professionals can be an essential part of an individual's support network and can work together with patients to develop a comprehensive treatment plan.

Support Groups

Support groups can offer a sense of community and understanding for individuals with bullous pemphigoid. Support groups can provide a safe space for individuals to share their experiences, offer advice, and provide emotional support. Support groups can also offer information about the condition and provide guidance on managing symptoms and navigating the healthcare system.

Tips for Building a Support Network for Bullous Pemphigoid

Building a support network for bullous pemphigoid requires time, effort, and an open mind. Here are some tips for building and maintaining a support network:

1. Identify Potential Support Resources: Start by identifying potential sources of support, including family members, friends, healthcare professionals, and support groups.

2. Communicate Your Needs: Let your support network know what kind of support you need, whether it is emotional support, practical assistance, or information about the condition.

3. Join a Support Group: Consider joining a support group dedicated to individuals with bullous pemphigoid. Support groups can offer a sense of community and understanding.

4. Be Open to New Relationships: Be open to building new relationships with individuals who share similar experiences or interests.

5. Prioritize Self-Care: Make time for self-care activities that promote physical and emotional well-being.

6. Stay Positive: Focus on the positive aspects of life and the support network that surrounds you.

Incorporating a Support Network into Daily Life

Incorporating a support network into daily life requires intentional effort and planning. Patients with bullous pemphigoid can schedule regular check-ins with family and friends or attend support group meetings as part of their routine. Patients can also communicate regularly with healthcare professionals and seek their guidance and advice as needed. Additionally, patients can prioritize self-care activities, such as exercise or meditation, as a way to build resilience and maintain overall well-being.

Communicating with healthcare professionals

Effective communication with healthcare professionals is crucial for individuals with bullous pemphigoid to receive optimal care and manage their condition effectively. In this article, we will discuss the importance of communicating with healthcare professionals and offer tips for effective communication.

The Importance of Communicating with Healthcare Professionals for Bullous Pemphigoid

Bullous pemphigoid is a chronic autoimmune disorder that requires ongoing medical treatment and management. Effective communication with healthcare professionals is essential for individuals with bullous pemphigoid to receive the best possible care. Good communication can help individuals receive a timely diagnosis, better manage their symptoms, and develop a comprehensive treatment plan.

Tips for Communicating with Healthcare Professionals for Bullous Pemphigoid

Here are some tips for effective communication with healthcare professionals when managing bullous pemphigoid:

1. Be Prepared: Before attending an appointment, prepare a list of questions, concerns, or symptoms you want to discuss with the healthcare professional. This can help ensure that you address all your concerns and make the most of your appointment.

2. Share Your Complete Medical History: Be sure to share your complete medical history, including any past illnesses, surgeries, or medications you have taken. This information can help the healthcare professional better understand your overall health and develop a treatment plan tailored to your needs.

3. Be Honest and Open: Be honest and open with the healthcare professional about your symptoms, including their severity and frequency. This information can help the healthcare professional better understand your condition and develop an appropriate treatment plan.

4. Ask Questions: Don't be afraid to ask questions about your condition, treatment options, and any concerns you may have. Asking questions can help you better understand your condition and make informed decisions about your healthcare.

5. Seek Clarification: If you don't understand something the healthcare professional says, ask for clarification. This can help ensure that you have a clear understanding of your condition and treatment plan.

6. Be Proactive: Take an active role in your healthcare by following the treatment plan recommended by the healthcare professional, scheduling regular appointments, and keeping track of your symptoms.

7. Communicate Changes in Your Condition: If you experience any changes in your condition or symptoms, let your healthcare professional know as soon as possible. This can help them make any necessary adjustments to your treatment plan.

Chapter Eight

Bullous Pemphigoid in Special Populations

Bullous pemphigoid is an autoimmune disease that can affect people of all ages, genders, and ethnicities. However, the disease can present unique challenges and complications in certain special populations. In this article, we will discuss how bullous pemphigoid affects special populations and the unique considerations that healthcare professionals need to take into account when treating these populations.

Bullous Pemphigoid in the Elderly

Bullous pemphigoid is more common in older adults, with the majority of cases occurring in people over 60 years old. The disease can present unique challenges in this population due to the increased likelihood of comorbidities, polypharmacy, and decreased immune function.

Older adults with bullous pemphigoid may be more susceptible to infection, which can worsen their symptoms and increase their risk of complications. Healthcare professionals need to monitor these patients closely for infections and adjust their treatment plans accordingly.

Additionally, many older adults with bullous pemphigoid may be taking multiple medications for other health conditions. Healthcare professionals need to be aware of potential drug interactions and adjust medication doses and schedules as needed.

Bullous Pemphigoid in Pregnancy

Bullous pemphigoid is rare in pregnant women, but when it does occur, it can present unique challenges for both the mother and the fetus. In some cases, bullous pemphigoid can lead to preterm labor, low birth weight, and fetal distress.

Treatment of bullous pemphigoid during pregnancy can be challenging due to concerns about the safety of certain medications for the developing fetus. Healthcare professionals need to carefully consider the risks and benefits of each treatment option and work closely with the patient to develop a treatment plan that is safe and effective.

Bullous Pemphigoid in Children

Bullous pemphigoid is rare in children, but when it does occur, it can present unique challenges due to the child's smaller size and developing immune system.

Children with bullous pemphigoid may require lower doses of medication than adults due to their smaller size. Additionally, healthcare professionals need to carefully monitor children for side effects and adjust treatment plans as needed.

Bullous Pemphigoid in People with Chronic Kidney Disease

Bullous pemphigoid can present unique challenges in people with chronic kidney disease due to the increased risk of infection and the potential impact of kidney disease on medication metabolism and excretion.

Healthcare professionals need to closely monitor people with chronic kidney disease for infections and adjust treatment plans as needed. Additionally, medication doses may need to be adjusted based on kidney function, and certain medications may need to be avoided altogether.

Bullous Pemphigoid in People with HIV/AIDS

Bullous pemphigoid can occur in people with HIV/AIDS, and the disease can present unique challenges in this population due to the impact of HIV/AIDS on the immune system and the increased risk of opportunistic infections.

Treatment of bullous pemphigoid in people with HIV/AIDS may require the use of different medications and treatment regimens than in the general population. Additionally, healthcare professionals need to closely monitor these patients for infections and adjust treatment plans as needed.

Pediatric

cases

Bullous Pemphigoid (BP) is a rare, autoimmune skin disease that primarily affects older adults. However, pediatric cases of BP have also been reported, albeit less frequently. In children, BP is often more severe and can lead to significant morbidity. Below we will explore the characteristics of BP in children, including its epidemiology, clinical features, diagnosis, and treatment options.

Epidemiology

BP is a relatively rare disease, and its prevalence in children is even lower. The incidence of BP in children is estimated to be less than 1 case per million per year. BP is more common in adults, with a peak incidence in individuals over the age of 60. The disease affects both genders equally, and there is no racial or ethnic predilection.

Clinical Features

BP in children presents similarly to the adult form of the disease, with the appearance of tense blisters and urticarial plaques on the skin. However, the clinical features of BP in children can differ from those seen in adults. For example, children with BP are more likely to develop widespread skin involvement, including the scalp, face, neck, and trunk. In contrast, BP in adults tends to involve the lower extremities more commonly. Additionally, children with BP are more likely to have oral involvement, which can result in difficulty eating or drinking.

The severity of BP in children can vary widely, ranging from mild blistering to severe, life-threatening disease. The clinical course of the disease can also be more aggressive in children than in adults, with rapid progression and a higher risk of relapse.

Diagnosis

The diagnosis of BP in children is based on clinical presentation, histopathology, and direct immunofluorescence (DIF) testing. Histopathology typically reveals subepidermal blistering with eosinophilic infiltrates. DIF testing shows linear IgG and C3 deposits at the basement membrane zone. Serological testing can also be performed, but it is less reliable in children than in adults.

It is important to differentiate BP from other blistering disorders, such as epidermolysis bullosa, pemphigus, and dermatitis herpetiformis, which can present similarly to BP. A skin biopsy with histopathology and DIF testing is necessary to make an accurate diagnosis.

Treatment

The treatment of BP in children is similar to that in adults and involves the use of topical and systemic therapies. Topical corticosteroids are often the first line of treatment, and they can be used in combination with oral corticosteroids, such as prednisone, in more severe cases. Other systemic therapies, such as azathioprine, mycophenolate mofetil, and rituximab, may also be used, but their efficacy and safety in children have not been well established.

The use of intravenous immunoglobulin (IVIG) has been reported as an effective treatment option in severe cases of BP in children. IVIG works by modulating the immune system and reducing inflammation. It is typically reserved for cases that are refractory to other treatments or in cases where corticosteroids are contraindicated.

Pregnancy and bullous pemphigoid

Bullous pemphigoid is a rare autoimmune disorder characterized by blistering and inflammation of the skin and mucous membranes. Although it is more commonly diagnosed in older adults, it can also affect pregnant women. Below we will explore the relationship between pregnancy and bullous pemphigoid, including its prevalence, potential causes, diagnosis, and treatment.

Prevalence

Bullous pemphigoid is a rare disease that affects approximately 1-2 people per 100,000 in the general population. It is even rarer in pregnant women, with only a few reported cases in the medical literature. However, studies suggest that pregnancy can be a triggering factor for the onset of bullous pemphigoid, and women with a history of the disease may experience a flare-up during pregnancy.

Causes

The exact cause of bullous pemphigoid is unknown, but it is believed to be an autoimmune disorder in which the body's immune system mistakenly attacks the skin and mucous membranes. During pregnancy, the immune system undergoes significant changes to prevent rejection of the developing fetus. This shift in immune function can sometimes trigger autoimmune disorders or cause existing autoimmune diseases to worsen.

Diagnosis

Diagnosing bullous pemphigoid during pregnancy can be challenging because the symptoms of the disease are similar to those of other skin conditions that commonly occur during pregnancy, such as pruritic urticarial papules and plaques of pregnancy (PUPPP). However, if a pregnant woman presents with blisters, erosions, or ulcers on the skin or mucous membranes, a skin biopsy and blood tests may be performed to confirm the diagnosis. It is important to note that the safety of skin biopsy during pregnancy has not been well studied, and the risks and benefits should be carefully considered before the procedure is performed.

Treatment

The treatment of bullous pemphigoid in pregnant women is similar to that in non-pregnant individuals, with the primary goal being to control the symptoms and prevent complications. Topical or systemic corticosteroids are typically the first-line treatment for bullous pemphigoid. However, the use of systemic corticosteroids during pregnancy is associated with an increased risk of gestational diabetes, preeclampsia, premature delivery, and low birth weight. Therefore, the dosage and duration of corticosteroid therapy should be carefully monitored.

In cases where corticosteroids are not effective or cannot be used, other immunosuppressive medications, such as azathioprine or mycophenolate mofetil, may be considered. However, these medications should be used with caution during pregnancy due to the potential risk of birth defects and other adverse outcomes.

In rare cases, plasmapheresis or intravenous immunoglobulin (IVIG) may be used to manage severe cases of bullous pemphigoid. However, the safety of these treatments during pregnancy has not been well established, and the risks and benefits should be carefully weighed before they are used.

Elderly patients

Bullous pemphigoid (BP) is an autoimmune disorder that primarily affects elderly individuals. As the world's population ages, the prevalence of BP is expected to rise, making it crucial to understand how the disease manifests in this population and how it can be treated effectively. Below we will explore the unique challenges of diagnosing and treating BP in elderly patients and discuss strategies for managing the disease in this population.

Symptoms of BP in elderly patients may be atypical or nonspecific, which can make diagnosis challenging. For example, elderly patients with BP may present with pruritus, or severe itching, without the classic blisters that are typically associated with the disease. Additionally, other comorbidities such as diabetes, hypertension, and renal disease may mask or exacerbate symptoms of BP, leading to delayed or misdiagnosis. In some cases, BP may also be mistaken for other dermatological conditions such as herpes zoster, pemphigus, and drug eruptions.

To diagnose BP in elderly patients, dermatologists typically perform a skin biopsy, which involves taking a small sample of skin tissue to examine under a microscope. Blood tests may also be conducted to detect the presence of antibodies associated with BP. However, as elderly patients may be more fragile, careful consideration must be given to the risk of biopsy-associated complications, such as bleeding and infection.

Treatment of BP in elderly patients may be complicated by the presence of other medical conditions and medications. For example, corticosteroids, which are commonly used to suppress the immune system and reduce inflammation in BP, may worsen pre-existing conditions such as diabetes and hypertension. Alternative therapies, such as topical steroids, may be preferred in some cases. Additionally, medication dosages may need to be adjusted or medications may need to be changed altogether to avoid drug interactions.

It is also important to monitor elderly patients for potential side effects of treatment, such as osteoporosis, cataracts, and infections. Regular bone density scans and eye exams may be recommended to catch and manage these potential complications early.

In addition to medical treatment, elderly patients with BP may benefit from lifestyle changes that support their overall health and well-being. This may include regular exercise, a healthy diet, and stress management techniques such as meditation or yoga. For elderly patients who may struggle with mobility, physical therapy or occupational therapy may also be beneficial.

Finally, it is important to provide emotional support to elderly patients with BP, as the disease can be distressing and impact their quality of life. Support groups or counseling services may be helpful in managing the emotional impact of the disease and connecting patients with others who are experiencing similar challenges.

Chapter Nine

The Future of Bullous Pemphigoid Research

Bullous pemphigoid (BP) is a rare autoimmune disorder that causes blistering and lesions on the skin and mucous membranes. While the exact cause of BP is still not completely understood, researchers continue to investigate possible triggers and treatment options. The future of BP research looks promising as new therapies are being developed and existing treatments are being refined.

One area of research is focused on identifying biomarkers that may predict disease severity and help guide treatment decisions. Several studies have looked at the levels of certain proteins and enzymes in the blood and skin of BP patients to determine if they can serve as biomarkers. Additionally, genetic studies are exploring the role of specific genes in the development and progression of BP.

Another area of research is focused on developing more targeted therapies for BP. Current treatments, such as corticosteroids and immunosuppressive medications, can have significant side effects and may not be effective for all patients. Researchers are exploring the use of biologics, which are drugs that target specific molecules involved in the immune response. Biologics have shown promising results in clinical trials for other autoimmune disorders, and may hold potential for treating BP.

Research is also being conducted on the role of the gut microbiome in autoimmune disorders, including BP. The gut microbiome is a collection of bacteria and other microorganisms that live in the digestive tract and play a role in immune system function. Studies have shown that imbalances in the gut microbiome can contribute to the development and progression of autoimmune disorders. Researchers are exploring the use of probiotics and other interventions to modulate the gut microbiome and potentially improve outcomes for BP patients.

Advances in technology are also shaping the future of BP research. For example, advances in imaging techniques, such as confocal microscopy, allow for non-invasive visualization of skin and mucous membrane lesions, which can aid in diagnosis and monitoring of disease activity. Additionally, machine learning and artificial intelligence are being used to analyze large data sets of patient information and identify patterns and predictors of disease progression.

While much progress has been made in understanding BP and developing treatments, there is still much work to be done. Research is ongoing to identify new therapies, improve existing treatments, and better understand the underlying mechanisms of BP. Through collaborative efforts between researchers, clinicians, and patients, the future of BP research looks promising for improving outcomes and quality of life for those living with this rare autoimmune disorder.

Advances in diagnosis and treatment

Bullous pemphigoid (BP) is a rare autoimmune disease that primarily affects older adults. It is characterized by the formation of fluid-filled blisters on the skin and mucous membranes, which can be accompanied by itching and burning sensations. The current standard of care for BP involves the use of systemic corticosteroids and immunosuppressive medications, but these treatments can cause significant side effects and may not be effective for all patients. As such, there is a need for continued research into more targeted and effective therapies for this disease.

One area of promising research involves the development of new diagnostic tests for BP. Currently, the gold standard for diagnosis is a skin biopsy followed by immunofluorescence testing to detect the presence of autoantibodies. However, these tests can be time-consuming and may not be readily available in all healthcare settings. Researchers are exploring the use of blood tests and other non-invasive diagnostic tools to improve the accuracy and accessibility of BP diagnosis.

In addition to improving diagnosis, there is ongoing research into more targeted and effective treatments for BP. One approach involves the use of biologic medications, which are designed to specifically target the immune system components involved in the disease. For example, some studies have shown promising results with the use of rituximab, a monoclonal antibody that targets B cells, which play a key role in the autoimmune response that leads to BP. Other biologic agents, such as omalizumab and dupilumab, are being studied for their potential to target specific inflammatory pathways involved in the disease.

Another area of research focuses on the use of topical treatments for BP. While systemic medications are effective for many patients, they can cause significant side effects and may not be well-tolerated in elderly or immuno compromised individuals. Topical therapies, such as high-potency corticosteroids and immunomodulators, may offer a safer and more targeted approach to managing the disease in some patients.

Finally, there is ongoing research into the underlying causes of BP and the genetic and environmental factors that may increase an individual's risk for developing the disease. This research may lead to new insights into the pathogenesis of BP and the development of more effective preventative measures.

Promising therapies

Bullous pemphigoid is an autoimmune disorder characterized by the formation of fluid-filled blisters on the skin. While traditional treatments for bullous pemphigoid, such as corticosteroids and immunosuppressants, have shown some success, researchers are actively exploring new therapies that may offer more targeted and effective treatments for this condition.

One promising area of research involves the use of biologic drugs that target specific immune system pathways involved in the development of bullous pemphigoid. For example, some studies have explored the use of drugs that target interleukin-17 (IL-17), a pro-inflammatory cytokine that has been implicated in the development of bullous pemphigoid. Other biologic agents that have shown promise in the treatment of bullous pemphigoid include rituximab, which targets B cells, and omalizumab, which targets IgE.

In addition to biologic therapies, researchers are also investigating the use of topical treatments for bullous pemphigoid. One example is the use of topical rapamycin, a drug that has been shown to inhibit the activation of T cells and reduce inflammation in the skin. Other topical treatments that have been explored for bullous pemphigoid include tacrolimus, pimecrolimus, and nicotinamide.

Gene therapy is another area of research that may hold promise for the treatment of bullous pemphigoid. Some studies have explored the use of gene therapy to deliver specific genes to the skin, with the goal of promoting the growth of healthy skin cells and reducing inflammation. While still in the early stages of development, gene therapy may eventually offer a targeted and long-lasting treatment for bullous pemphigoid.

Beyond these specific therapies, researchers are also exploring the potential benefits of a range of supportive interventions for individuals with bullous pemphigoid. These may include nutritional supplements to support skin health, such as vitamin D and omega-3 fatty acids, as well as lifestyle interventions like stress reduction techniques and exercise programs.

Despite the promising advances in research on bullous pemphigoid, much work remains to be done in order to develop effective and accessible treatments for this condition. However, with continued research and innovation, there is hope that individuals living with bullous pemphigoid may one day have access to a wider range of effective treatments and supportive interventions to manage their symptoms and improve their quality of life.

Clinical trials and ongoing research

Bullous pemphigoid (BP) is a chronic autoimmune disease that affects the skin and mucous membranes. Although there are treatments available, there is still a need for further research and development of therapies to improve the quality of life for patients with BP. Clinical trials and ongoing research are essential to advancing the understanding and treatment of BP.

Clinical trials are research studies that involve human participants to test the effectiveness and safety of new medications, treatments, and procedures. Clinical trials for BP are essential to identify new therapies and improve existing treatments. These trials can provide important data about the efficacy and safety of potential treatments, which can then be further studied in larger trials or potentially approved for use by regulatory agencies.

There are currently several clinical trials underway to investigate new therapies for BP. One example is a Phase 2 clinical trial testing the effectiveness of a medication called rituximab. Rituximab is a monoclonal antibody that targets specific immune cells involved in the development of BP. This trial is designed to evaluate the safety and effectiveness of rituximab in treating BP and is expected to conclude in 2023.

Another clinical trial currently underway is investigating the use of a medication called omalizumab. Omalizumab is a monoclonal antibody that targets specific proteins involved in the immune response. This trial is designed to evaluate the safety and effectiveness of omalizumab in treating BP and is expected to conclude in 2024.

Ongoing research into the pathophysiology of BP is also critical to the development of new therapies. Researchers are investigating the molecular and cellular mechanisms that lead to the development of BP to identify potential targets for new therapies. For example, studies have shown that certain immune cells, called T cells, play a crucial role in the development of BP. Targeting these cells could potentially be a promising therapeutic approach.

Additionally, researchers are investigating the potential use of gene therapy in the treatment of BP. Gene therapy involves introducing new genetic material into cells to correct or replace faulty genes. This approach could potentially be used to target the specific immune cells involved in the development of BP, providing a more targeted and effective therapy.

Furthermore, advancements in diagnostic techniques and tools are also essential for improving the diagnosis and treatment of BP. For example, researchers are exploring the use of biomarkers, such as specific antibodies or genetic markers, to aid in the diagnosis and monitoring of BP. Improved imaging techniques, such as high-resolution ultrasound and confocal microscopy, can also aid in the diagnosis and monitoring of BP by allowing for more accurate visualization of the affected skin and mucous membranes.

Chapter Ten

Resources and Support

Bullous Pemphigoid (BP) is a rare, chronic autoimmune disorder that affects the skin and mucous membranes. It causes the formation of fluid-filled blisters or bullae that appear on the skin, typically in the groin, armpits, and other skin folds. BP primarily affects older adults, and it is estimated to affect around 1 in 40,000 people annually. While there is no known cure for BP, there are various treatment options available that can help manage the symptoms of the condition.

Individuals living with BP may require support and resources to help them cope with the condition. Below we will explore some of the resources and support available for those living with BP.

Support Groups:

Support groups can be a valuable resource for individuals living with BP. These groups provide a safe and supportive environment for individuals to share their experiences, connect with others who have similar experiences, and receive emotional support. Support groups can be found through local hospitals, community centers, or online.

National Organizations:

National organizations can provide a wealth of information and resources for individuals living with BP. These organizations offer educational materials, advocacy and support, and access to clinical trials and research studies. The International Pemphigus & Pemphigoid Foundation (IPPF) is a leading national organization for pemphigoid patients. The IPPF offers a variety of resources, including a peer support program, educational webinars, and an annual patient conference.

Patient Education:

Education is key to understanding BP and managing its symptoms. Patients can seek education from their healthcare providers or by accessing educational materials online. The IPPF provides educational resources for patients and healthcare providers. Additionally, the American Academy of Dermatology (AAD) offers patient education materials on BP, including symptoms, diagnosis, and treatment options.

Mental Health Support:

Living with a chronic condition like BP can take a toll on mental health. It is essential for individuals with BP to seek mental health support when needed. This can include talking to a mental health professional, joining a support group, or seeking peer support. The IPPF offers a peer support program that connects individuals with trained volunteers who have experienced the condition.

Financial Assistance:

Living with a chronic condition like BP can be expensive. Treatment costs, medications, and other expenses can quickly add up. There are resources available to help individuals with the financial burden of living with a chronic condition. The National Organization for Rare Disorders (NORD) offers financial assistance programs for individuals with rare diseases, including pemphigoid.

Clinical Trials:

Clinical trials offer individuals with BP access to new and potentially more effective treatment options. These trials test new treatments and therapies, and individuals may be able to participate in clinical trials through their healthcare providers. The IPPF maintains a database of current clinical trials for pemphigoid patients.

Organizations and foundations

Bullous Pemphigoid is a rare autoimmune disorder that affects the skin, causing blistering and lesions on the surface. Coping with this condition can be overwhelming, which is why it's important to have access to resources and support. Fortunately, there are several organizations and foundations dedicated to providing assistance to individuals and families affected by Bullous Pemphigoid.

One such organization is the International Pemphigus and Pemphigoid Foundation (IPPF). This non-profit organization offers a wide range of resources and support services to those living with Bullous Pemphigoid and other pemphigus and pemphigoid diseases. The IPPF offers a free information packet, a patient support hotline, educational materials, and opportunities to connect with others through online support groups and regional events. The organization also offers research grants to fund studies aimed at improving the diagnosis and treatment of pemphigus and pemphigoid diseases.

The National Organization for Rare Disorders (NORD) is another valuable resource for individuals and families affected by Bullous Pemphigoid. NORD is a patient advocacy organization that offers information about rare diseases, patient assistance programs, and support services. The organization also provides educational materials and resources for healthcare professionals to improve diagnosis and treatment options for rare diseases.

The American Autoimmune Related Diseases Association (AARDA) is a non-profit organization dedicated to increasing awareness and understanding of autoimmune diseases. The organization provides educational resources, conducts research, and advocates for improved public policies related to autoimmune diseases. The AARDA also offers support groups, a patient education and advocacy program, and an autoimmune disease research program.

In addition to these organizations, there are also online support groups and forums where individuals and families can connect with others who are living with Bullous Pemphigoid. These groups provide a sense of community and offer a platform for sharing experiences, resources, and support.

It's important to note that finding the right resources and support is a personal decision, and what works for one person may not work for another. It's essential to explore all available options and find the resources and support that best meet your needs.

In addition to these organizations, there are also several ways to manage the psychological impact of living with Bullous Pemphigoid. Mental health professionals, such as therapists and counselors, can provide support and guidance for coping with the emotional challenges of living with a chronic illness. Mindfulness and relaxation techniques, such as yoga and meditation, may also help reduce stress and improve overall well-being.

Online communities

Bullous pemphigoid is a rare autoimmune disorder that affects the skin, causing blistering and inflammation. It can be a difficult condition to manage, both physically and emotionally. However, connecting with others who have the same condition can help make it easier to cope. One way to do this is through online communities.

There are several online communities dedicated to bullous pemphigoid, where individuals with the condition can connect, share information and experiences, and offer support to one another. These communities may take the form of discussion forums, social media groups, or online support groups.

One such community is the International Pemphigus & Pemphigoid Foundation (IPPF), which has an online support group specifically for individuals with bullous pemphigoid. The IPPF is a non-profit organization that provides education, support, and advocacy for individuals affected by pemphigus and pemphigoid. Their online support group is a private forum where members can ask questions, share their experiences, and offer support to others in the community.

Another online community for individuals with bullous pemphigoid is the Daily Strength Support Group. This group is a public forum where members can share their experiences and connect with others who have the same condition. Members can also create their own discussion threads on specific topics related to bullous pemphigoid, such as treatment options or coping strategies.

In addition to these larger communities, there may also be smaller, more niche groups for individuals with specific needs or interests. For example, some groups may focus on managing the condition during pregnancy, while others may be geared towards individuals who have been recently diagnosed. These smaller groups can provide a more intimate setting for individuals to connect and share information with others who have similar experiences.

Online communities can offer several benefits for individuals with bullous pemphigoid. Firstly, they provide a platform for individuals to connect with others who have the same condition, which can be a source of comfort and support. Secondly, they can provide valuable information on treatment options, coping strategies, and other aspects of managing the condition. Finally, they can help combat feelings of isolation and loneliness that can come with living with a rare condition.

However, it is important to remember that not all information found online is accurate or trustworthy. It is essential to verify the information with a healthcare professional before acting on it. Additionally, while online communities can provide support and information, they should not replace medical advice or treatment.

Educational materials and tools

Bullous pemphigoid is a rare autoimmune disorder that causes painful blisters to form on the skin. It is a chronic condition that can be difficult to manage, but with the right education and tools, patients can learn to effectively manage their symptoms and improve their quality of life.

One of the most important aspects of managing bullous pemphigoid is educating patients about the condition and its treatments. Educational materials can take many forms, including brochures, websites, and videos. These materials should be easy to understand and provide clear information about the causes, symptoms, and treatments of bullous pemphigoid.

There are many resources available to patients with bullous pemphigoid. These resources can include support groups, online forums, and educational websites. Patients can also access information about their condition through their healthcare provider, who can provide educational materials and answer questions about the condition and its treatments.

One useful tool for patients with bullous pemphigoid is a symptom tracker. Symptom trackers allow patients to record information about their symptoms, including the location and severity of their blisters, and any changes they notice over time. This can help patients and their healthcare providers track the progress of the disease and make informed decisions about treatment.

Another tool that can be helpful for patients with bullous pemphigoid is a treatment plan. A treatment plan outlines the specific steps that patients should take to manage their symptoms, including medications, topical treatments, and lifestyle changes. It can also include information about how to recognize and manage potential side effects of treatment.

In addition to educational materials and tools, patients with bullous pemphigoid can benefit from the support of their healthcare providers, family, and friends. Patients should be encouraged to discuss their condition with their healthcare providers and seek support from friends and family. They may also find it helpful to join a support group or online forum, where they can connect with others who are living with the same condition.

* 9 7 8 1 7 7 6 9 6 7 9 8 8 *
SD - #0222 - 070926 - C0 - 229/152/5 - PB - 9781776967988 - Matt Lamination